The Ultimate Guide to Losing Weight the Healthy Way

Detox Your Body, Improve Your Health and Eat Well

70+ Delicious Alkaline Recipes to Reset and Rebalance

Creative Spun

TABLE OF CONTENT

interim quality. Trademarks that are mentioned are done without written consent and can in no way be considered an endorsement from the trademark holder.

Introduction

Having a healthy diet makes your life in many ways. Almost anyone looking to better their life can follow this diet. Unhealthy eating has become prominent all over the world. People of all ages prefer to run away from vegetables and fruits these days practically.

Apart from some popular ingredients, people don't know about the large variety of available foods at their disposal. Because of laziness and ignorance, people choose not to look at all of the options that might greatly benefit them and settle for the most comfortable thing they can get on the plate. Dieting, especially alkaline dieting, is a crucial step in improving people's health because it focuses mainly on vegetables and fruits.

The diet effectively makes a person lose weight and reach their weight goals, so obese and overweight people can significantly improve their lives. Also, it can help people suffering from heart disease and diabetes. Learn how you can lose weight the healthy way in this book. Let's go through it together.

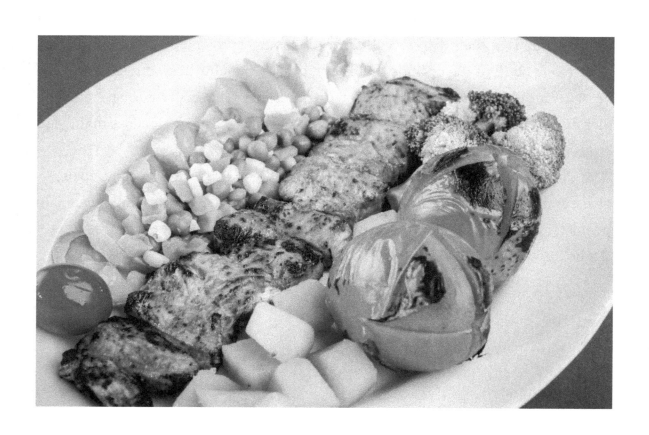

CHAPTER 1

WHAT EXACTLY IS THE ALKALINE DIET?

A good diet is a change in one's regular lifestyle that does not only restrict the intake of harmful food in general but to live a healthier, longer and disease-free life.

The diet, also called the alkaline diet, is a plant-based diet developed by the late . It's claimed to rejuvenate your cells by eliminating toxic waste by alkalizing your blood. The diet relies on eating a list of approved foods along with many supplements.

Alfredo Bowman (late), popularly referred to as, is a self-proclaimed herbalist and Honduran who uses food to enhance health. He has claimed to cure many diseases using herbs and a strict vegan diet due to his holistic approach. Although he calls himself, he doesn't hold any medical nor Ph.D. degree. However, he claimed to have used this diet to cure different conditions like sickle-cell anaemia, lupus, leukemia, and HIV-AIDS.

This led to several controversies, particularly that he was practicing medicine without a license and making outrageous claims. While he was charged for practicing without a license, he was acquitted within the early 1990s due to a lack of evidence. However, he was instructed to stop making claims that his diet can treat HIV-AIDS. While there are controversies that surround his name, there are numerous benefits of his alkaline vegan diet.

THE ALKALINE DIET

An alkaline diet assumes that certain products, such as berries, vegetables, roots, and legumes, leave an alkaline residue or ash behind in the body. The body is strengthened by rock's key ingredients, such as calcium, magnesium, titanium, zinc, and copper. To avoid chronic diseases such as asthma, malnutrition, exhaustion, and even cancer, an alkaline diet is the perfect prevention tool.

It is believed that acidity and mucus could cause different types of diseases. For instance, the build-up of mucus in the lungs can lead to pneumonia. It was acclaimed that eating certain types of food and avoiding others like the plague can help detoxify the body. It can also bring the body to an alkaline state that can reduce the risk of developing many diseases. By turning the blood alkaline, the cells can be rejuvenated and can quickly eliminate toxins out. Moreover, it was proclaimed that conditions could not exist in an environment that is alkaline. This principle of making the body more alkaline is what other plant-based diets are banking on.

The plan, which requires a stringent nutritional regime and supplements, promises to detoxify the body and restore alkalinity. The diet restricts any animal products and focuses on vegan plant-based foods but with much more stringent rules. It is essentially a raw vegan diet that does not focus on portion control but instead on consuming the right food. emphasized that this diet should be followed consistently for the rest of your life. It might seem quite restrictive, but there are some delicious recipes on the diet that will make you forget the highly refined, processed food you are used to.

The Diet is plant-based, but unlike other plant-based diets, there are some differences in this diet to the plant-based diet in general. Here is a compiled list of what differentiates the Diet from a plant-based diet.

1. **No processed foods:** Tofu, veggie burgers, textured vegetable protein, canned fruits, canned vegetables, oil, soy sauce, and other condiments are considered processed. The diet encourages dieters to consume unadulterated food. Some plant-based diets still allow processed foods as long as they are made from plant-based ingredients.

2. **No wheat products allowed:** Under this diet regimen, you are not allowed to consume wheat and wheat products such as bread, biscuits, and others as they are not naturally growing grains. Naturally growing grains include amaranth seeds, wild rice, and triticale, to name a few. The need to adhere to the food list: In general, plant-based diets are not so restrictive when it comes to the food that dieters are allowed to eat (unless you are explicitly following a strict plant-based regimen such as the plant-based keto diet). However, the diet requires dieters only to eat foods listed in the nutritional guide.

3. **Drink one gallon of water daily:** Water is the most hydrating liquid on the planet. The diet requires dieters to consume 1 gallon of water daily or more. Moreover, tea and coffee should be avoided as these drinks are highly acidic.

4. **Taking in supplements**: If you are taking any medications for a particular health condition, this particular diet regimen will require you to consume proprietary supplements an hour before taking your medication.

Almost anyone looking to better their life can follow this diet. Unhealthy eating has become prominent all over the world. People of all ages prefer to run away from vegetables and fruits these days practically. Apart from some popular ingredients, people don't know about the large variety of available foods at their disposal. Because of laziness and ignorance, people choose not to look at all of the options that might greatly benefit them and settle for the most comfortable thing they can get on the plate. Dieting, especially alkaline dieting, is a crucial step in improving people's health because it focuses mainly on vegetables and fruits.

Those who will benefit most from this diet are are obese people looking to shed some pounds so that they don't invite diseases into their bodies. The diet effectively makes a person lose weight and reach their weight goals, so obese and overweight people can significantly improve their lives. Also, it can help people suffering from heart disease and diabetes.

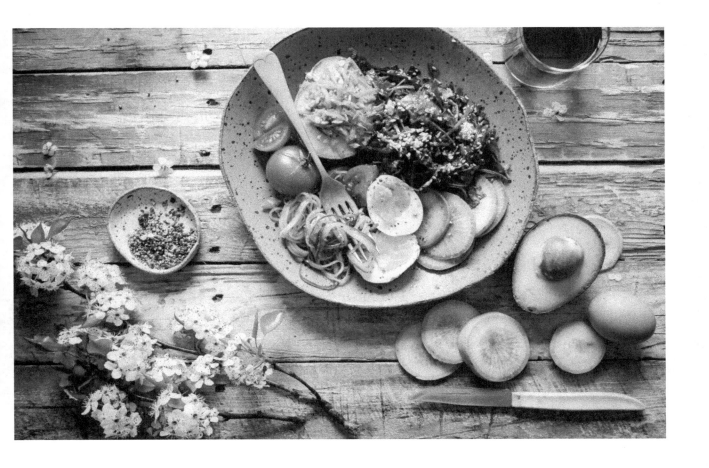

HOW TO START ALKALINE DIET

Before diving into the essential tips required for starting an Alkaline Diet, let talk about why food is vital to the human body, how it is processed, and the concept of metabolism.

Why is food so important?

Every human being needs food to live, to have the power to work, to fight harmful elements, to revitalize cells and tissues, and to eliminate toxins from the body. Finding the right food has always been a problem for humans. The earliest inhabitants of the Earth only used a vegetarian diet. Over time, they began to hunt and fish. When they discovered fire, people began to vary their diet; now, they had the tools to cultivate and raise animals. In the 19th century, refined products like sugar, flour, and other concentrates became common products. In the 20th century, people started to use hybrid and genetically modified foods due to selective breeding and reproduction by mutations.

We need food to get the fat, protein, vitamins, minerals, and carbohydrates that our bodies need every day to synthesize nutrients. With the help of digestion, we can obtain essential enzymes, amino acids, and other nutrients essential for the functioning of our body. They will keep us healthy and strong. With the help of metabolism, we get the most out of nutrients. Simply put, the faster our cells, tissues, and organs synthesize small molecules, the fitter our body stays.

Digestion

Digestion is a form of catabolism that helps us break down large food molecules into small soluble molecules absorbed through the small intestines into the bloodstream and then into the cells, tissues, and organs.

The digestive system starts with chewing. The contact of food with the saliva starts the digestion and provides the ideal conditions of pH. The processed food travels to the stomach, wherewith the aid of gastric acids and enzymes, it is transformed into smaller molecules. After a few hours, the resulting liquid enters the duodenum, where, with the assistance of pancreatic digestive enzymes and bile juice from the liver, it continues to be digested. Once digestion is over, the nutrients are absorbed into the blood. So, proteins are converted to amino acids, glucides to glucose, and lipids to fatty acids.

Metabolism

The metabolism is a set of chemical reactions in any organism. It helps us convert the essential nutrients from foods into energy converse foods into proteins, nucleic acids, lipids, and carbohydrates and also eliminate the nitrogenous waste

TIPS FOR STARTING THE DIET

Mindset

Having a positive mindset is the most crucial tool needed for starting the Diet. The nutritional guide for Diet is quite restrictive, some ingredients are not that easy to find in any supermarket, but with a bit of patience, you will come to realize that it is not that hard. Mindset is essential, as in anything worth fighting for; when you want to lose weight, you must consider that restriction is a must, and obstacles will always pop up when least expected. Try to focus on your goal and not on how limited your meal options are.

Being emotionally ready is a big step ahead. Although changing your eating habits is not easy, daily habits are firmly inserted into our subconscious, so we must take the time to adjust them. Begin with small steps and keep telling yourself that this is the right way to achieve your goals, weight loss, and overall health. Get support from your family and friends, surround yourself with positive people, and proceed step-by-step. Small changes each day will lead to lifetime healthy eating habits.

Listed below are some of the acts to adopt when opting to start 's Diet.

Drink water

Water is probably our body's most important (after oxygen) resource. Hydration in the body is vital as the water content determines the body's chemistry. The body contains approximately 55% to 78% of water, depending on the body's size and age. People tend to survive without food for a month but can't last more than a few days without water. Water plays a significant role in maintaining the human brain and ensures the body's proper functioning by cleansing and eliminating various toxins from the body.

These supplements contain herbs that promote urination to remove toxins from the body. So, one must drink more water to replenish the water eliminated. You are advised to drink up to one gallon of water a day to keep the body well hydrated. Springwater is his best choice since it is naturally alkaline. Tap water and other sources of water may contain high levels of chloride and other contaminants.

Avoid acidic drinks like Tea, coffee, or soda

Our body also attempts to regulate the acid and alkaline content. There is no need to consume carbonated drinks as the body refuses carbon dioxide as a waste.

Breathe

Oxygen explains that our body works, and if you provide the body with adequate oxygen, it should perform better. Sit back and enjoy two to five minutes of slow breaths. Nothing is easier than you can perform Yoga.

Avoid packaged food and food with artificial sweeteners

The reason to avoid packaged and processed foods is that our body has not been programmed to absorb preservatives and sweeteners. These sweeteners, which tend to be high in low fat, are potentially detrimental to the body. Besides, Saccharin, a primary ingredient in sweeteners, triggers cancer. Keep away from these things.

Exercise

The alkaline and the acidic element will also be matched. This is not just a question of taking in alkaline milk. A little acid (because of muscles) often regulates natural bodywork.

Avoid Snacks

Satiate your urges for a snack by eating vegetables or soaked nuts - Whenever we are thirsty, we still consume a little fast food. Establish a tradition of consuming fresh vegetables or almonds, even walnuts.

Sleep well

Seek to escape the pain. Our mind regulates the digestive system, and only when in a relaxed, focused condition can you realize it functions appropriately. Relax, then, and remain safe!

HEALTH BENEFITS OF ALKALINE DIET

There is no medical data to endorse the lifestyle of dieting. Research suggests, however, that a diet focused on plants will improve wellbeing. Some of the health benefits of the diet include;

Weight Reduction in a healthy manner

Limiting your intake of acidifying foods and eating more alkaline foods can protect your body from obesity by reducing leptin levels and inflammation, which affects your hunger and your ability to burn fat. Since alkaline foods are anti-inflammatory, an alkaline diet allows your body to achieve normal levels of leptin and feel satisfied eating the number of calories it needs.

Weight reduction is one of the main reasons to adopt 's alkaline diet. The diet is based on consuming vegetables and fruits, which are high in vitamins, minerals, fiber, and other compounds associated with reduced inflammation, oxidative stress, and protection against many diseases. A study has shown that those who ate seven or more servings of fruits and vegetables a day had a lower incidence of cancer and heart disease. This diet is based on principles opposite to the Western diet since it restricts us from processed foods, dense fats, sugar, salt, and other harmful ingredients.

Boost Immune System

Maintaining an alkaline body directly relates to our health and well-being. However, staying alkaline isn't always easy. The human body can become too acidic by consuming processed foods, environmental stressors, medications, too much sugar, and too much caffeine, which makes us more vulnerable to disease and illness. An alkaline diet is a simple and effective way to avoid these stressors.

Flooding your cells with immune-boosting alkaline foods reduces inflammation, balances your pH, and strengthens your immune system.

Higher life expectancy

A major anti-aging effect of an alkaline diet is that it reduces inflammation and increases growth and hormone production. It has been shown to improve cardiovascular health and protect against common problems such as high cholesterol, hypertension (high blood pressure), kidney stones, strokes, and even memory loss. Alkaline diets have been proven to help prevent plaque buildup in blood vessels, stop calcium buildup in urine, strengthen bones, prevent kidney stones, reduce muscle wasting or spasms, which prolongs the lifespan.

Prevents Disease

The buildup of body acid waste (or acidosis) is a primary cause of virtually every documented illness, including (but not only) diabetes, obesity, liver disease, renal disease, coronary disorder, neurologic disease, premature ageing, hormonal imbalances, osteoporosis, and also the majority of cancers. Degenerative diseases flourish in acidic conditions, and they may be stripped of their capacity to replicate or even take root by destroying their ideal climate.

An extract published in the Journal of Environmental and Public Health in 2012 notes that a diet rich in alkaline foods doesn't only prevent kidney disease but leads to increased levels of growth hormone. It helps prevent muscle wasting and can even help treat chronic pains and inflammation. A 2016 study in Alternative Therapies in Health and Medicine confirms this improvement in bone mineral density and muscle mass. This study also suggests that consuming alkaline food and water can reduce tumor cell growth and metastasis, effectively remove toxins from the body, and reduce the incidence of cardiovascular disease. If you decide to keep your body free of disease, safe and robust, follow an alkaline diet and enjoy a healthy life.

Greater Energy and Increased Muscle Mass.

The further fluids that accumulate inside the body, the less effectively the body's normal balance processes will handle, which might increase the body's acidity. The greater the acid levels, the more alkaline elements (calcium, magnesium, phosphates, etc.) are extracted from the skin, muscles, and tissue to ensure that the blood retains the requisite alkaline content to ensure the body works. If the useful synthesis of these alkaline minerals is impaired, it contributes to leniency and exhaustion. The leaching of these minerals was often correlated with osteoporosis. If the amounts of acid are lowered by proper nutrition and exercise, energy rates should increase.

Following an alkaline diet can help maintain muscle mass as you age, an important factor in preventing falls and fractures. A three-year clinical trial involving 384 men and women (65 years and older) published in the American Journal of Clinical Nutrition in 2008 determined that a high intake of foods high in potassium, such as the recommended fruits and vegetables, can help older people maintain lean muscle mass as they age.

Body Detoxification.

By strictly following this diet and using these proprietary and expensive supplements, the promise is to restore your body's natural alkaline state and detoxify your diseased body.

HOW THE ALKALINE DIET CAN BENEFIT THE ELDERS ABOVE 50 YEARS

The alkaline diet is known to provide many health advantages, but I would particularly like to explore this diet's bonuses for individuals in their golden era. Why do we consider the alkaline diet to be particularly beneficial in the golden years of people? Part of the explanation is that the work of the kidney decreases with age. Because the kidneys are responsible for removing acidic substances from diets, older adults may be vulnerable to a low-alkaline diet's harmful consequences.

The most significant adverse impact I like to think about is bone degradation. The most severe bone condition is osteoporosis, as the body attempts to deal with the development of superfluous acid by withdrawing alkaline minerals from the bones. Nonetheless, at the risk of long-term bone degradation, this briefly prevents the internal condition from being highly acidic. Luckily, you may avoid this by following a safe, nutritious diet. The tissues will break down to release alkaline minerals like your teeth. Therefore, it is not shocking that excess acidity is involved in wasting tissue. And at least one analysis suggests that eating more alkaline diets will support muscle tissue in older adults.

A healthy diet can help avoid any of the worst aspects of growing older with daily exercise and an optimistic mindset. The health issues which many people find "natural" are the product of an unhealthy lifestyle instead. The positive news is that if an issue emerges from a deficiency, a balanced alkaline diet will overcome it.

CHAPTER 2

ALKALINE'S APPROACH TO DISEASE

Some of the chronic diseases we can cure with 's diet include:

Obesity

Obesity is a chronic disease where the accumulated excess body fat leads to a variety of conditions such as type 2 diabetes, cardiovascular disease, obstructive sleep apnea, osteoarthritis, depression, and even some types of cancer. It is caused by poor eating habits, an inactive lifestyle, genetics, gut flora, mental illness, and social determinants. The best cure for obesity is to eat fruits and vegetables, stay away from meat and alcohol, and drink a lot.

Herpes and STDs

Herpes and all STDs are viral infections that cannot be overcome by the immune system. STDs can be only be prevented by having Safe sex. 's cure for Herpes and STDs includes herbal teas such as burdock and dandelion, eating plenty of dates and lettuce.

Hypertension/ High blood pressure.

Hypertension is a long-term health problem where blood pressure is consistently high. It is a major risk factor for stroke, vision loss, heart failure, and even dementia. For healing, one should stay away from meat and alcohol, drink too much tea, and eat fruits and vegetables approved by. Vegetables to eat include olives, wild rice, lettuce, cucumber, bell pepper, kale, squash, valerian, and chickpeas. Dried fruits are the best choice for our diet.

Stress ulcer

A stomach ulcer is a discontinuity in the body membrane that interferes with the normal functioning of the affected organ. The stress ulcer is the most common type of ulcer in all countries. It mainly affects the stomach and can lead to ulcerative gastritis, stricture, and massive bleeding. 's remedy includes consuming vegetables like tomatoes and squash, ripe fruits (apples, peaches, raisins), sour soups, and lots of herbal teas, especially fennel and chamomile, for their calming effect.

Type-2 diabetes

It is a chronic disease that occurs as a result of obesity, especially in people over the age of 40. It is characterized by a lack of insulin, a crucial factor for digestion. To cure diabetes, we must avoid fried foods, tea with sugar, rice, and lentils. Vegetables to be eaten include kale, cucumber, lettuce, cherry tomatoes and plums, chickpeas, bell pepper, squash, mushrooms, dandelion, and onions. We can only eat fruits such as red raspberries, plums, apples, and limes without stones. Sour soups are highly indicated for the treatment of type 2 diabetes.

Constipation

Constipation is a condition that has a profound impact on our well-being. Abdominal pain, bloating, and irregular bowel movements can lead to other complications, such as hemorrhoids and anal fissures. 's remedy is to eat fruits (mainly apples, peaches, plums, figs), vegetables (pumpkin, kale, and chickpeas), basil, nuts, and lots of herbal teas, especially the fennel, dandelion, and chamomile.

Atherosclerosis

Atherosclerosis occurs when the arteries become narrow and can lead to strokes, coronary artery disease, and kidney problems. It is prohibited to smoke and consume alcohol. Coffee should be limited, but lettuce tea is a real help. In addition to exercise, we should eat wild rice, fruits, and vegetables.

Gout

Gout is inflammatory arthritis characterized by severe recurring pain, red, hot, and swollen joints due to low levels of uric acid in the blood. It can lead to kidney disease. In this case, we have to combine the fiber with the uric acid in the digestive tract so that it no longer forms crystalline deposits. The most reliable way to prevent gout is to lose weight, get plenty of vitamins, and avoid alcohol. According to specialists, food supplements have no effect on gout, but advises us to drink burdock, dandelion, and elderberry tea. Eating alkaline fruits and vegetables also helps reduce uric acid levels.

Asthma

This occurs as an effect of the chronic inflammation of the lungs caused by an excessive accumulation of mucus, environmental and genetic causes. It's quite difficult to prevent it but easier to cure. Traditional medicine uses vitamins, fatty acids, breathing maneuvers, and breathing techniques to keep the lungs functioning properly. recommends that we use fennel, anise, chamomile tea, and alkaline fruits and vegetables.

GERD (gastroesophageal reflux disease)

GERD is a long-term disorder in which the contents of the stomach move up into the esophagus. The main cause is insufficient closure of the esophageal sphincter, but obesity, obstructive sleep apnea, and gallstones are also involved. We need to change our lifestyle, eat healthily, start exercising, quit smoking, and permanently give up acidic foods. This is why 's nutritional guide will help us overcome this condition.

HOW DOES THE ALKALINE DIET ASSIST WITH CANCER

Have you ever been curious why the heart never got cancer? Although the heart can potentially be damaged by cancer like some other part of the body, we rarely hear about heart cancer. This is because the heart is rarely cancerous. An alkaline diet can be the only effective way to prevent cancer and to get rid of it. Let us consider what cancer induces and how an alkaline diet can avoid it.

When tossing contaminants, every cell in our bodies absorbs oxygen, nutrients, and glucose. The immune system defends these cells. Yet, the immune response becomes overwhelmed by contaminants, and the cell cannot consume oxygen and eventually ferments when the tissue becomes acidic. The cell is damaged by cancer and is destroyed. The next issue is cancer avoidance and treatment by having less acidic than an alkaline diet. The solution to cancer, therefore, resides in a highly alkaline diet. With the right intake contributing to a high alkaline pH, cancer cells cannot survive in this setting.

Anaerobic cancer cells cannot exist in oxygen. We can survive even under low levels of oxygen. When an alkaline diet preserves the pH of the body, the body's immune system maintains high. This causes cells to obtain ample oxygen and to remove their toxic waste. In these conditions, cancer can neither grow nor take life.

ALKALINE PLANT FOOD AND HERBS

Alkaline Plant Food

Most alkaline plant Food can be considered superfood not only for their capacity to help our body uphold a healthy pH balance but also for their nutrient density. The most alkaline foods are usually plant-based and have multiple healing properties. Listed below are some alkalizing foods, all of which are delicious and versatile.

1. **Tomatoes:** They are most alkaline when they are uncooked but comprise many nutrients, raw and uncooked. Tomatoes are excellent sources of digestive enzymes, vitamin C, and a good source of vitamin B6, which is often hard to find. It is advisable to consume sliced tomatoes as a snack with a bit of pink sea

salt or mix them into your desired salad, omelet, and other varieties of food.

2.   Almonds: Almonds are a great alkaline snack or addition to any recipe. They are high in healthy fats, which makes them satiating and nutritious. The high magnesium content of almonds makes them alkaline.

3. Spinach: Most green leafy vegetables are alkaline in the body, but spinach is one of our favorites because it is very versatile. Even those who don't like vegetables will often appreciate spinach for its mild flavor. It is rich in chlorophyll, vitamin K, vitamin A, and many more. Always try to add spinach to your morning green smoothie or mix them into your desired salad and omelet.

4.   Parsley: It is a very alkalizing food that's also outstanding at cleansing the kidneys and supporting the digestive system. It can be consumed parsley in juice or as a nutrient-dense ingredient in many different dishes, from soups to chilis to salads!

5.   Lemon: Lemons are known to be one of the most alkalizing foods. They are great for healthy detox, aid digestion, and help the liver flush toxins from the body. Drinking a glass of lemon water every morning is a great habit that should be part of your daily routine. It will help you feel good all day.

6.   Jalapeno: Not only are Jalapenos alkaline-forming but most peppers, mild to spicy and helps our bodies maintain a healthy pH level. To those who enjoy a punch, jalapenos are a fantastic addition to an alkaline diet, it helps support the endocrine system and also prevent free radicals in the body.

7.   Garlic: Garlic is an anti-inflammatory food that ranks very high on the alkaline scale. Garlic has been shown to prevent disease, boost immunity, and act as a powerful antibacterial agent in our system.

8.   Avocado: It is a powerhouse of both nutrients and deliciousness. Avocado contains a lot of healthy fats and is also alkalizing, anti-inflammatory, and heart-healthy.

9.   Basil: Basil is one of our favorite alkalizing ingredients. High in vitamin A, K & calcium, basil also has a high concentration of flavonoids, which have antioxidant properties.

10. Red Onion: Cooking onions lightly can increase the alkalinity of onions, but consuming them raw is also a fantastic choice, as onions have a variety of nutritional benefits in addition to alkaline properties. Onions are rich in vitamin C and have anti-inflammatory and antibacterial effects.

11. Green Leafy Vegetables: Many leafy greens have an alkaline influence on our bodies. They include minerals that are important for the body to perform various functions. Seek to eat broccoli, cabbage, celery, arugula, and mustard greens.

12. Cauliflower and Broccoli: They're perfect enough for you whether you enjoy broccoli sautéed in Asian spices or gobi matar. It includes some essential phytochemicals for the body. Take it with other vegetables such as capsicum, rice, and green peas, and there you have your dose of food.

13. Citrus Fruits: Unlike the misconception that citrus fruits are highly acidic and poisonous to the body, they are the best alkaline food source. Citrus fruits, lime, and oranges are filled with Vitamin C, which is believed to consistently help to detoxify the body by acid reduction and heart-burning.

14. Seaweed and Sea Salt: Were you conscious that seaweed or marine vegetables are 10-12 times higher than those cultivated on land? These are often considered too alkaline types of food and provide multiple benefits for the body's function. It would be best to introduce it into your soup or stir-fries bowl or create sushi at home. And dust the greens, soups, omelettes, etc., with sea salt.

15. Root Vegetables: Root crops such as sweet potatoes, taro root, lotus root, beets, and carrots are excellent alkali sources. You eat better when grilled with a mix of spices and other seasonings. They're always overcooked, and they miss all their beauty. Be patient when cooking and enjoy root vegetables as you know to use them in soups, fried meats, salads, and more.

16. Seasonal Fruits: Any nutritionist and fitness professional will inform you that you will benefit from incorporating seasonal fruit into your everyday diet. Seasonal fruits are filled with vitamins, minerals, and antioxidants that take charge of various body functions. They are also good sources of alkaline nutrition, especially kiwi, pineapple, persimmon, nectarine, watermelon, grapefruit, apricots, and apples.

17. Onion, Garlic, and Ginger: In Indian cuisine, onion, garlic, and ginger are essential ingredients. They are used and consumed in various forms. Garlic can be used to dust the morning bread, ginger in the broth or tea and onions in salads, etc.

ALKALINE HERBS

Boosting your body's alkalinity with herbs is as easy as sipping a tea. Some of the herbs recommended by and their respective uses include:

1.   Cascara Sagrada: is a shrub plant that most people only know as a "dietary supplement" and was allowed to be sold in pharmacies as over the counter drugs. However, in 2002, FDA declared that it doesn't meet the standards to be sold as over-the-counter drugs (OTC) or prescription drugs. Before then, the dietary supplement or Cascara Sagrada's bark was used as a purgative for constipation. One sweet thing about this shrub is that it is a bitter less extract that can also be used as a flavoring agent.

2.   **Rhubarb Root**: is the root and underground stem (that is, rhizome) of the Rhubarb plant. The traditional Chinese people have used this plant's root as a medication to treat digestive tract disorders, including stomach pain, constipation, menstrual cramps (dysmenorrhea), diarrhea, and swelling of the pancreas, etc. This plant's stems are also used as a flavoring agent and mostly used to make a pie and serve as great recipes. Because of this root's chemical content, such as fiber, research has it that it is a potent laxative. It has the potency to reduce swelling, treat cold sores, improve the digestive tract stone and health, cleanse heavy metal and harmful bacteria. It also enhances the general movement of the intestines and reduces cholesterol levels.

3.   **Prodigiosa:** is also known as the 'Brickellia Grandiflora herb.' It is a flowering plant/shrub from the daisy family and native to Mexico and California. The Mexican has used these plants/shrubs as a tea to treat diarrhea, diabetes, and stomach pain. Research carried on Prodigiosa shows that the plant is an antioxidant, it contains chemical compounds that aid in stimulating the pancreatic gland to secret and reduces or lowers blood sugar level, aid the digestion of fat in the gallbladder, and also improve the healthiness of the stomach digestive system.

4. **Burdock root**: is the root of a plant called Burdock that can be found worldwide. Virtually everything about Burdock is essential as its root is used as food and medicine, and its leaf and seed are used for medicinal purposes. Many people believe that consuming Burdock helps increase urine flow, eradicate germs, purify the blood, prevent and treat cancer, joint pain, cold, diabetes, anorexia, fever, bladder infections, syphilis, stomach, and intestinal complaints. This plant does not stop there as it also helps treat and prevent skin diseases such as; acne and psoriasis. Burdock also boosts sex drive (libido), lowering high blood pressure and cleansing of the liver and lymphatic system.

5. **Dandelion:** is a flowering plant known as "Taraxacum officinale." It is native to Europe. It is commonly found in the mild climates of the northern hemisphere. These flowering plants have been used for centuries before now for the treatment of swelling (inflammation) of the pancreas, cancer, tonsils (tonsillitis), acne, bladder or urethra, digestive, and liver disorders. Because of the vitamin (A, B, C, E, and K), mineral (iron, potassium, magnesium, and calcium), and other compounds (Polyphenols, Chicoric and Chlorogenic acid) that Dandelion contains, research has it that it has the potency to detoxify gallbladder, kidney and purifies the blood. It also dissolves kidney stones, treats and prevents diabetes, and relieves liver and urinary disorders. It also contains chemicals that may increase urine production, which helps in cleansing the urinary tract and prevent crystals from forming in the urine.

6.   **Elderberry**: is also known as European elderberry or black elder, or Sambucus nigra. This flowering plant belongs to the Adoxaceae family and is native to Europe. It is common in Europe and many other parts of the world. This plant can grow as long as 9 meters. It is 30feet tall and has many clusters (white or cream-colored flowers) known as elderflowers. The leaves of elderberry have been used for many years for the treatment of pain, inflammation, swelling, and to stimulate urine production, and induce sweat. The bark is not left behind as it was also used as a laxative, diuretic, and to induce vomiting.

7.   **Guaco**: is a climbing plant known as Guace or Vedolin or Cepu or Bejuco de Finca or Liane Francois or Cipo caatinga and other names. This climbing plant is rich in various minerals and compounds. It is from the family of Asteraceae and species of cordifolia. Its leaf is very medicinal and nutritional.

8.   **Mullein** is a flavorful beverage plant also known as Aaron's rod, Candlewick, American mullein, Adam's flannel, Dense Flowered mullein, Candleflower, European or orange mullein, etc. This flavorful beverage plant has been used for centuries before now to treat diverse sicknesses, including asthma, tuberculosis, pneumonia, chills, flu, gastrointestinal bleeding, colds, chronic coughs, and others.

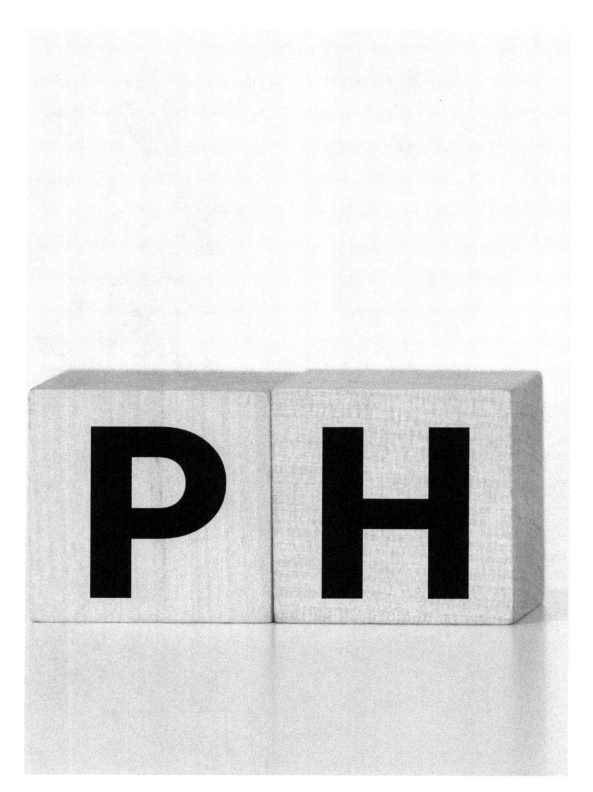

CHAPTER 3

THE DIFFERENCE BETWEEN BLOOD PH, SALIVA PH AND HOW TO MEASURE THEM

Blood pH

The abbreviation pH stands for potential hydrogen. It is used to describe chemical acidity in relation to the level of alkalinity of a substance. It ranges from 0 to 14. It measures the acidity of a solution of a substance in water. For instance, pure water has a pH of 7. Low pH solutions have a high concentration of hydrogen ions and are acidic. High pH solutions have a lower concentration of hydrogen ions and are alkaline or basic. Black coffee and vinegar are acidic and drop below a pH of 7. Antacids and seawater are alkaline and test above pH of 7. With a pH just above 7, the blood of a healthy human is somewhat alkaline.

Normal Blood pH levels

The pH of the blood in the arteries must be between 7.35 and 7.45 for the metabolic processes of the body and other systems to work properly. These metabolic processes produce acids, so the body has a complex feedback and regulation system to maintain a healthy pH level. Much of the acid produced in the body is carbon dioxide. This is formed when carbon dioxide combines with water. Carbon dioxide is produced in the tissues of the body as a result of the respiratory process.

The lungs and kidneys are the two main organs that regulate blood pH, often at the same time. There are also chemical buffering mechanisms in all cells of the body. The lungs can help to quickly regulate the blood pH by exhaling carbon dioxide, which sometimes causes changes within seconds. For example, when someone is exercising, they produce more carbon dioxide and breathe faster to the acidity of the body.

The kidneys regulate the pH of the blood by excreting acids in the urine. They also produce and regulate bicarbonate, which also increases the pH of the blood. These changes last longer than the changes that occur due to breathing and can last for hours or days.

Changes in the pH blood level

Certain medical situations and conditions can prevent the body from keeping the blood pH in a healthy state. The pH of the blood can either be too acidic or less acidic. When the blood is too acidic, this is called Acidosis, which is when the body has a pH below 7.35, while Alkalosis occurs when the blood is not acidic enough, that is when the body has a pH higher than 7.45. The various ways in which the blood pH can change:

1. **Metabolic acidosis**: This ensues as a result of reduced bicarbonate or increased acid levels.
2. **Respiratory acidosis**: This occurs when the body removes less carbon dioxide than usual.
3. **Metabolic alkalosis**: This occurs due to increased bicarbonate or reduced acid levels.

4. **Respiratory alkalosis**: This occurs when the body removes more carbon dioxide than usual.

Symptoms of blood pH changes

When a person's blood pH is above or below the healthy range, they begin to experience specific symptoms. Their symptoms will depend on whether their blood has become more acidic (acidosis) or is no longer acidic enough (alkalosis). Some of the symptoms of acidosis and alkalosis are listed below:

Symptoms of acidosis

1. Headache
2. Confusion
3. Tiredness
4. Lethargy and sleepiness
5. Coughing and shortness of breath
6. An uneven or increased heart rate
7. Stomach upset or feeling sick
8. Muscle seizures or weakness
9. Unconsciousness and coma

Symptoms of alkalosis

Common symptoms of alkalosis include having shaky hands, vomiting and nausea, numbness or tingling in the face, feet, and hands, prolonged muscle cramps, lightheadedness, etc.

How to measure blood pH.

Blood ph is measured by doing the blood gas test. A blood gas test provides an accurate measurement of the levels of oxygen and carbon dioxide in your body.

A small blood sample must be taken for a blood gas test. Arterial blood can be obtained from the veins in your wrist, arm, or groin or from a pre-existing arterial line if you are currently hospitalized. A blood gas sample can also be venous, from a vein or a pre-existing intravenous or capillary line, requiring a small heel prick.

The test measures the pH of arterial blood, which indicates the number of hydrogen ions in the blood. A pH below 7.0 is called acidic, and a pH above 7.0 is called basic or alkaline. A lower blood pH can indicate that your blood is more acidic and has a higher carbon dioxide content. A higher blood pH may indicate that your blood is more alkaline and has a higher bicarbonate content.

Saliva pH.

The standard pH range for saliva is 6.2-7.6. Food and drink change the pH of saliva. For instance, bacteria in your mouth break down the carbohydrates you eat, which releases lactic acid, butyric acid, and aspartic acid, which indirectly lowers the pH level of your saliva. However, age is one of the factors that influence the pH level of your saliva. Children tend to have less acidic saliva than adults.

Why care about the pH of my saliva?

The mouth needs a balanced pH like the rest of your body. The pH of your saliva can drop below 5.5 when you drink acidic drinks. As a result of this, the acids in your mouth start to demineralize (break down) the tooth enamel. If tooth enamel becomes too thin, dentin is exposed. This can cause discomfort when consuming hot, cold, or sugary drinks.

Here are some examples of acidic foods and drinks:

- Soft drinks (pH 3).
- White wine (pH 4).
- American cheese (pH 5).
- Cherries (pH 4).

Symptoms of unbalanced saliva pH

Some of the symptoms that indicate changes in your saliva pH are:

1. Insistent bad breath.
2. High sensitivity to hot food, cold food, or beverages.
3. Tooth cavities.

How to keep a balanced pH in my mouth?

To maintain a balanced pH in your mouth, you should only consume foods and drinks with an average pH. However, that would be pretty boring and likely rob you of essential minerals and vitamins. A more acceptable idea would be to modify your behavior with certain foods and drinks, such as:

1. Avoid sugary sodas: But if you can't resist the temptation, Drink adequate water after consuming them but try not to drink sugary drinks for long periods.

2. Avoid black coffee: Adding dairy products, not a sugar-flavored cream, can help counteract heartburn.

3. Don't brush: Don't brush your teeth immediately after drinking high acid beverages, such as soda, fruit juices, cider, wine, or beer. High acid drinks soften the tooth enamel. Brushing immediately after consuming these drinks can further damage enamel.

4. Bubble gum: Chew sugar-free gum after eating or drinking acidic foods or drinks, preferably one with xylitol. Chewing gum stimulates saliva production to help restore the pH balance. Xylitol is believed to prevent bacteria from adhering to tooth enamel; it also stimulates the production of saliva.

5. Keep hydrated: Drink lots of water with pH seven.

How to measure Saliva pH.

To test your saliva's pH, you'll need pH strips. It can be bought online or at any drug store nearby. Having purchased the pH strip, you can follow these steps:

1. Avoid the intake of any food or drinks for a minimum of two hours before performing the test.

2. Fill your mouth with saliva and swallow or spit.

3. Refill your mouth with saliva and place a small amount on a pH strip.

4. The strip will change color depending on the acidity/alkalinity of your saliva. The outside of the box of pH strips has a color chart. Match the

color of your pH strip to the color chart to determine the pH level of your saliva.

Difference between Blood pH and Saliva pH

pH indicates the level of H + ions, with a low pH indicating too many H + ions and a high pH indicating too many OH ions. The pH of blood ranges from 7.35 to 7.45, while the pH of saliva ranges from 6.5 to 7.5. After ingestion, the food travels to the stomach, where the upper and lower parts of the stomach have different pH levels. The top part has a pH of 4 to 6.5, while the bottom part has a pH of 1.5 - 4.0 (very acidic). It then enters the slightly alkaline intestine, with a pH of 7 to 8.5 for digestion. Maintaining the pH levels of different regions is essential to their function.

CHAPTER 4

MISCONCEPTIONS WHEN YOU ARE INTO PLANT-BASED DIET

Misconceptions 1: Plant-based diets are high in carbohydrates that raise blood sugar levels

FACT: There are different types of carbohydrates. Carbohydrates can be refined or unrefined. Refined and highly processed carbohydrates, such as those found in candy, table sugar, syrups, soda, and flour, break down quickly and are absorbed by the body, causing blood sugar to rise. In contrast, unrefined carbohydrates found in most fruits and vegetables take longer to digest, and sugar is released into the bloodstream more slowly. Many studies suggest that people with diabetes can improve their blood glucose control by switching to a completely plant-based diet

Misconception 2: "A Plant-Based Diet is Too Time Consuming."

Still, preparing whole foods, even fresh and healthy, doesn't have to mean hours in the kitchen. Vegetables like broccoli and squash can be steamed in minutes, and salads can be cut, spun, mixed, and eaten quickly. Many consumers create a weekly menu and fill their freezer with the food they can eat all week, meaning a plant-based diet doesn't require more time, just better planning.

Eating whole foods and plant-based diets may take more time than always microwaving a frozen meal, but there is plenty of whole food and frozen foods. Edlong flavors are an excellent, easy way to ensure ready-to-eat foods are packed with the authentic taste consumers expect.

Misconception 3: You get hungry faster after eating plant-based meals.

FACT: Plants are generally lower in calorie density than meat products, so it is rational to assume that the first does not fill the stomach like the second. Still, whole foods are high in fiber, a plant-based macronutrient crucial for digestion. Individuals who consume large amounts of fiber are more likely to feel full longer than those who do not because it cannot be easily broken down. These macronutrients are only found in fruits, vegetables, whole grains, and legumes, so be sure to eat the recommended amount of plant foods every day. It has also been shown to have several other benefits, including maintaining blood sugar and lowering cholesterol.

Misconception 4: Plant-based diets are nutritionally poor

FACT: A diet rich in vegetables, fruits, legumes, whole grains, nuts, and seeds is very nutritious. Aside from serving as a beautiful source of disease-fighting antioxidants and fiber, plant foods also provide healthy levels of protein and calcium. Citrus fruits are significantly rich in vitamin C, while leafy vegetables are rich in calcium, iron, and zinc. Some vegetables even contain protein, ensuring that people get most, if not all, of the necessary amino acids and vitamins by consuming only plants. The major nutrients obtained from animal sources are vitamin B12, and vitamin D. People who eat little or no meat should consume vitamin B12. Vitamin D is produced in the skin after sun exposure, but if sun exposure is less than 5 to 15 minutes, people with dark skin or colder climates may need to take supplements or fortified foods (cereals, bread, milk, vegetables).

Misconception 5: Plant-based diet is expensive and difficult to prepare

FACT: Beans, grains, sweet potatoes, lentils, and fruits are plant-based foods that can be found in most local grocery stores at a relatively low cost and are covered by the Supplemental Nutrition Assistance Program (SNAP) benefits. Since plant-based meals use whole foods in their natural state, they often require fewer steps to prepare. The spices that you use in your favorite dishes, especially cultural dishes, can also be used to prepare vegetables and other whole foods. 100% plant-based foods cost much less than controlling diseases caused by poor nutrition. The costs of paying a caregiver, traveling to and from the doctor's office, lost wages, prescriptions, and copay go far beyond the cost of buying healthy foods.

Misconception 6: It's impossible to get enough protein on a plant-based diet

FACT: This is one of the biggest misconceptions when it comes to a plant-based diet. People tend to associate meat with protein, so a meat-free diet equates to a protein-free diet. In fact, consuming all the necessary proteins and amino acids in a plant-based diet can be more challenging but not impossible. While meat is one of the best-known forms of protein, protein isn't limited to just meat-based products. Beans, tofu, and nuts are the most common plant protein sources, but many vegetables like spinach and asparagus also contain protein. The recommended daily amount of protein is equal to 0.8 grams per kilogram of body weight, which is not difficult to achieve by consuming only plant products.

Misconception 7: Plant-based diets are not appropriate for people with kidney failure

FACT: New research suggests that a healthy plant-based diet can extend the lives of people with chronic kidney disease (CKD). Patients with CKD who consumed more plant protein than animal protein were less likely to die from the disease. However, patients with kidney disease should consult their doctor or dietitian to make sure they are getting the right nutrients in safe amounts, as dialysis puts them at risk for protein deficiency and high potassium and phosphorus levels in the blood.

Misconception 8: Eating Soy Increases Risk of Cancer

Fact: Contrary to the general belief, Soy does not increase the risk of breast cancer, it can actually help reduce it. Soy is a rich source of plant protein. Although soy has been a staple in the East Asian diet for centuries, there is a myth that overeating soy can increase the risk of breast cancer. However, experts from the American Cancer Society claim that soy is completely safe for both women and men. "So far, the research does not point to the dangers of consuming soy in humans, and the health benefits seem to outweigh the potential risks. There is growing evidence that consuming traditional soy products such as tofu, tempeh, edamame, miso, and soy milk may decrease the risk of breast cancer, especially in women. Soy products are great sources of protein, especially when replacing other less healthy foods such as animal fat and red or processed meat. Consuming Soy products have been linked to helping in reducing heart disease and may even help lower cholesterol. "

Misconception 9: Plant-Based foods are limited

Fact: There is a misconception that plant-based foods are boring and limited to smoothies in salads; this is false. By committing yourself to eat more fruits, vegetables, legumes, and grains, you're opening yourself up to thousands of new ingredients and flavors. Plant-based eating isn't limiting; it's limitless.

CHAPTER 5

LIST OF RECOMMENDED RECIPES

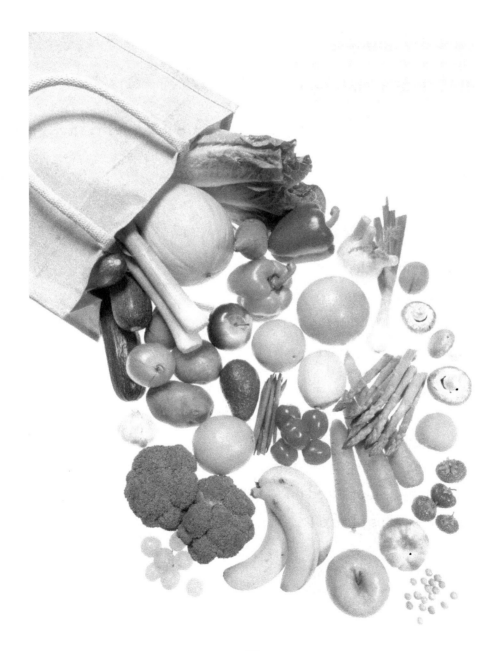

Vegetables

1. **Power Pesto Zoodles**

Servings: 2

Cooking time: 5 minutes;

Preparation time: 10 minutes;

Nutritional Info: 214 Cal; 1017.10 g Fats; 4.8 g Protein; 13.2 g Carb; 6.1 g Fiber;

Ingredients:

- 2 zucchini
- 1 avocado, peeled, pitted
- ½ cup cherry tomatoes
- 2 tablespoons walnuts
- ½ of key lime, juiced

Extra:

- ¼ teaspoon salt
- 1/8 teaspoon cayenne pepper
- 2 teaspoons grapeseed oil
- 2 tablespoons olive oil

Directions

1. Prepare the zucchini noodles and for this, cut them into thin strips by using a vegetable peeler or use a spiralizer.
2. Then take a medium skillet pan, add oil in it and when hot, add zucchini noodles in it and then cook for 3 to 5 minutes until a tender crisp is achieved.
3. Transfer the remaining ingredients into a food processor, then pulse until the creamy paste comes together.
4. When zucchini noodles have sautéed, drain and place them in a large bowl and add the blended sauce in it.
5. Add 2 tablespoons of water and then toss until well combined.
6. Garnish the zoodles with grated coconut and then serve.

2. Mushroom Gravy

Serving: 2

Cooking time: 12 minutes;

Preparation time: 5 minutes;

Nutritional Info: 65.3 Cal; 1.6 g Fats; 3.5 g Protein; 9.6 g Carb; 1 g Fiber;

Ingredients:

- ¾ tablespoon of spelt flour
- ¼ of onion, peeled, diced
- 4 ounces sliced mushrooms
- ½ cup walnut milk, homemade
- 1 tablespoon chopped walnuts

Extra:

- ¼ teaspoon salt
- 1/8 teaspoon cayenne pepper
- ½ teaspoon dried thyme
- 1 tablespoon grapeseed oil
- ¼ cup vegetable broth, homemade

Directions

1. Take a medium skillet pan, place it over medium heat, add oil and when hot, add onion and mushrooms, season with 1/16 teaspoon each of salt and cayenne pepper, and then cook for 4 minutes until tender.

2. Stir in spelt flour until coated, cook for 1 minute, slowly whisk in milk and vegetable broth and then season with remaining salt and cayenne pepper.

3. Switch heat to low-level, cook for 5 to 7 minutes until the sauce has thickened slightly and then stir in walnuts and thyme.

4. Serve straight away with spelt flour bread.

3.   Nori Burritos

Serving: 2

Cooking time: 0 minutes;

Preparation time: 10 minutes;

Nutritional Info: 90 Cal; 1.5 g Fats; 1.5 g Protein; 12.5 g Carb; 1 g Fiber;

Ingredients:

- 1 avocado, peeled, sliced
- 1 cucumber, deseeded, cut into round slices
- 1 zucchini, sliced
- 2 teaspoons sprouted hemp seeds
- 2 nori sheets

Extra:

- 1 tablespoon tahini butter
- 2 teaspoons sesame seeds

Directions

1. Working on one nori sheet at a time, place it on a cutting board shiny side down and then arrange half of each avocado, cucumber and zucchini slices and tahini on it, leaving 1-inch wide spice to the right.
2. Then start folding the sheet over the fillings from the edge that is closest to you, cut into thick slices, and then sprinkle with 1 teaspoon of sesame seeds.
3. Repeat with the remaining nori sheet, and then serve.

4. Zesty Citrus Salad

Serving: 2

Preparation time: 5 minutes; Cooking time: 0 minutes;

Nutritional Info: 265 Cal; 24 g Fats; 3.8 g Protein; 11.6 g Carb; 6.4 g Fiber;

Ingredients:

- 4 slices of onion
- ½ of avocado, peeled, pitted, sliced
- 4 ounces arugula
- 1 orange, zested, peeled, sliced
- 1 teaspoon agave syrup

Extra:

- 1/8 teaspoon salt
- 1/8 teaspoon cayenne pepper
- 2 tablespoons key lime juice
- 2 tablespoons olive oil

Directions

1. Distribute avocado, oranges, onion, and arugula between two plates.
2. Mix together oil, salt, cayenne pepper, agave syrup and lime juice in a small bowl and then stir until mixed.
3. Sprinkle the dressing over the salad and then serve.

5. Zucchini Hummus Wrap

Serving: 2

Cooking time: 8 minutes;

Preparation time: 10 minutes;

Nutritional Info: 264.5 Cal; 5.1 g Fats; 8.5 g Protein; 34.5 g Carb; 5 g Fiber;

Ingredients:

- ½ cup iceberg lettuce
- 1 zucchini, sliced
- 2 cherry tomatoes, sliced
- 2 spelt flour tortillas
- 4 tablespoons homemade hummus

Extra:

- ¼ teaspoon salt
- 1/8 teaspoon cayenne pepper
- 1 tablespoon grapeseed oil

Directions:

1. Take a grill pan, grease it oil and let it preheat over a medium-high heat setting.
2. Meanwhile, place zucchini slices in a large bowl, sprinkle with salt and cayenne pepper, drizzle with oil and then toss until coated.

3. Arrange zucchini slices on the grill pan and then cook for 2 to 3 minutes per side until developed grill marks.

4. Assemble tortillas and for this, heat the tortilla on the grill pan until warm and develop grill marks and spread 2 tablespoons of hummus over each tortilla.

5. Distribute grilled zucchini slices over the tortillas, top with lettuce and tomato slices, and then wrap tightly.

6. Serve straight away.

6.   Basil And Avocado Salad

Serving: 2

Cooking time: 0 minutes;

Preparation time: 10 minutes;

Nutritional Info: 387 Cal; 16.6 g Fats; 9.4 g Protein; 54.3 g Carb; 8.6 g Fiber;

Ingredients:

- ½ cup avocado, peeled, pitted, chopped
- ½ cup basil leaves
- ½ cup cherry tomatoes
- 2 cups cooked spelt noodles

Extra:

- 1 teaspoon agave syrup
- 1 tablespoon key lime juice
- 2 tablespoons olive oil

Directions

1. Take a large bowl, place pasta in it, add tomato, avocado, and basil in it and then stir until mixed.
2. Take a small bowl, add agave syrup and salt in it, pour in lime juice and olive oil, and then whisk until combined.
3. Pour lime juice mixture over pasta, toss until combined, and then serve.

7. Vegan Portobello Burgers

Serving: 2

Cooking time: 20 minutes

Preparation time: 10 minutes;

Nutritional Info: 354 Cal; 32.8 g Fats; 3.7 g Protein; 14.4 g Carb; 4.4 g Fiber;

Ingredients:

- 2 Portobello mushroom caps
- ½ of avocado, sliced
- 1 cup purslane
- 2 teaspoons dried basil
- 2 tablespoons olive oil

Extra:

- ¼ teaspoon salt
- 1 teaspoon dried oregano
- ½ teaspoon cayenne pepper

Directions

1. Switch on the oven, then set it to 425 degrees F and let it preheat.
2. Prepare the marinade and for this, take a small bowl, pour in oil, add cayenne pepper, onion powder, oregano, and basil and then stir until mixed.

3. Take a cookie sheet, line it with a foil, brush with oil, place mushroom caps on it, evenly pour the marinade over mushroom caps and then let them marinate for 10 minutes.

4. Then bake the mushroom caps for 20 minutes, flipping halfway, until tender and cooked.

5. When done, place mushroom caps on two plates, top the caps with avocado and purslane evenly and then serve.

8. Grilled Romaine Lettuce Salad

Serving: 2

Cooking time: 10 minutes;

Preparation time: 10 minutes;

Nutritional Info: 130 Cal; 2 g Fats; 2 g Protein; 24 g Carb; 4 g Fiber;

Ingredients:

- cut in half two small heads of romaine lettuce,
- 1 tablespoon chopped basil
- 1 tablespoon chopped red onion
- ¼ teaspoon onion powder
- ½ tablespoon agave syrup

Extra:

- ½ teaspoon salt
- ¼ teaspoon cayenne pepper
- 2 tablespoons olive oil
- 1 tablespoon key lime juice

Directions

1. Take a large skillet pan, place it over medium heat and when warmed, arrange lettuce heads in it, cut-side down, and then cook for 4 to 5 minutes per side until golden brown on both sides.

2. When done, transfer lettuce heads to a plate and then let them cool for 5 minutes.

3. Meanwhile, prepare the dressing and for this, place the remaining ingredients in a small bowl and then stir until combined.
4. Drizzle the dressing over lettuce heads and then serve.

9. Vegetable Fajitas

Serving: 2

Cooking time: 8 minutes;

Preparation time: 10 minutes;

Nutritional Info: 337 Cal; 3.7 g Fats; 2.6 g Protein; 73.3 g Carb; 21.3 g Fiber;

Ingredients:

- 2 Portobello mushroom caps, 1/3-inch sliced
- ¾ of red bell pepper, sliced
- ½ of onion, peeled, sliced
- ½ of key lime, juiced
- 2 spelt flour tortillas

Extra:

- 1/3 teaspoon salt
- ¼ teaspoon cayenne pepper
- ¼ teaspoon onion powder
- 1 tablespoon grapeseed oil

Directions

1. 4. Take a medium skillet pan, place it over medium heat, add oil and when hot, add onion and red pepper and then cook for 2 minutes until tender-crisp.

2. 5. Add mushrooms slices, sprinkle with all the seasoning, stir until mixed, and then cook for 5 minutes until vegetables turn soft.
3. 6. Heat the tortilla until warm, distribute vegetables in their center, drizzle with lime juice, and then roll tightly.
4. 7. Serve straight away.

10. Appetizing Baked Apple

Serving: 2

Cooking time: 55 minutes;

Preparation time: 10 minutes;

Nutritional Info: 346 Cal; 6.4 g Fats; 1.5 g Protein; 78 g Carb; 6.2 g Fiber;

Ingredients:

- 4 apples, large, cored, sliced
- 1/8 teaspoon ground cloves
- 3 tablespoons agave syrup
- 1 tablespoon chopped walnuts

Directions

1. Switch on the oven, then set it to 350 degrees F and let it preheat.
2. Meanwhile, take a large bowl, place apple slices in it, drizzle with agave syrup and then toss until evenly coated.
3. Take a small bowl, place nuts in it, add cloves, and then stir until mixed.
4. Sprinkle the nuts mixture over the apple and let it rest for 5 minutes or more until apples start releasing their juices.
5. Take a medium casserole dish, arrange apple slices on it, and then bake for 15 minutes.
6. Cover the casserole dish with foil and then continue baking for 40 minutes until bubbly.
7. Let apples cool for about 10 minutes and then serve.

11. Classic Banana Fries

Serving: 2

Cooking time: 10 minutes;

Preparation time: 5 minutes;

Nutritional Info: 130.5 Cal; 6.5 g Fats; 1 g Protein; 20 g Carb; 3 g Fiber;

Ingredients:

- 4 baby burro bananas, peeled, cut in squares
- ¼ teaspoon salt
- ½ of a medium onion, peeled, chopped
- ½ of medium green bell pepper, cored, chopped
- 2 teaspoons grapeseed oil
- ¼ teaspoon cayenne pepper

Directions

1. Take a medium skillet pan, place it over medium-low heat, add oil and when hot, add burro banana pieces and then cook for 3 minutes or until beginning to brown.
2. Then turn the burro banana pieces, add remaining ingredients, stir until mixed, and then continue cooking for 5 to 7 minutes until onions have caramelized.
3. Serve straight away.

12. Zoodles with Basil & Avocado

Serving: 2

Cooking time: 0 minutes;

Preparation time: 10 minutes;

Nutritional Info: 330 Cal; 20.7 g Fats; 7.1 g Protein; 35.3 g Carb; 7.8 g Fiber;

Ingredients:

- 2 zucchinis, spiralized into noodles
- 2 avocados, peeled, pitted
- ½ cup walnuts
- 2 cups basil leaves
- 24 cherry tomatoes, sliced

Extra:

- 1/3 teaspoon salt
- 4 tablespoons key lime juice
- ½ cup spring water

Directions

1. Prepare the sauce and for this, place all the ingredients except for zucchini noodles and tomatoes in a food processor and then pulse until smooth.
2. Take a large bowl, place zucchini noodles in it, add tomato slices, pour in the prepared sauce and then toss until coated.
3. Serve straight away.

13. Butternut Squash and Apple Burgers

Serving: 2

Cooking time: 1 hour;

Preparation time: 10 minutes;

Nutritional Info: 250 Cal; 4 g Fats; 6 g Protein; 51 g Carb; 5 g Fiber;

Ingredients:

- ¾ cup diced butternut squash
- ½ cup diced apples
- 1 cup cooked wild rice
- ¼ cup chopped shallots
- ½ tablespoon thyme

Extra:

- ¼ teaspoon sea salt, divided
- 1 tablespoon pumpkin seeds, unsalted
- 1 tablespoon grapeseed oil
- 2 spelt burgers, halved, toasted

Directions

1. Switch on the oven, then set it to 400 degrees F and let it preheat.
2. Meanwhile, take a cookie sheet, line it with a parchment sheet, spread squash pieces on it and then sprinkle with 1/8 teaspoon salt.
3. Bake the squash for 15 minutes, then add shallots and apple, sprinkle with remaining salt, and then bake for 20 to 30 minutes until cooked.

4. When done, let the vegetable mixture cool for 15 minutes, transfer it into a food processor, add thyme and then pulse until a chunky mixture comes together.

5. Add pumpkin seeds and cooked wild rice, pulse until combined, and then tip the mixture in a bowl.

6. Taste the mixture to adjust and then shape it into two patties.

7. Take a skillet pan, place it over medium heat, add oil and when hot, place patties in it and then cook for 5 to 7 minutes per side until browned.

8. Sandwich patties in burger buns and then serve.

14. Kale and "Avocado" Dish

Serving: 2

Preparation time: 5 minutes; Cooking time: 0 minutes;

Nutritional Info: 143 Cal; 10.5 g Fats; 3 g Protein; 12.4 g Carb; 4.8 g Fiber;

Ingredients:

- 1 bundle of kale, cut into thin strips
- 1 small white onion, peeled, chopped
- 12 cherry tomatoes, chopped
- 1 tablespoon salt
- 1 avocado, peeled, pitted, sliced

Directions

1. Take a large bowl, place kale strips in it, sprinkle with salt, and then massage for 2 mins.
2. Cover the bowl, then let it rest for a minimum of 30 minutes, and then pour and stir in onion and tomatoes until well combined.
3. Let the salad sit for 5 minutes, add avocado slices, and then serve.

15. Zucchini 'Bacon' Dish

Serving: 2

Cooking time: 20 minutes;

Preparation time: 10 minutes;

Nutritional Info: 184 Cal; 2 g Fats; 12 g Protein; 26 g Carb; 2 g Fiber;

Ingredients:

- 2 zucchini, cut into strips
- 1 tablespoon onion powder
- 1 tablespoon of sea salt
- ½ teaspoon cayenne powder

Extra:

- ¼ cup date sugar
- 2 tablespoons agave syrup
- 1 teaspoon liquid smoke
- ¼ cup spring water
- 1 tablespoon grapeseed oil

Directions

1. Take a medium saucepan, place it over medium heat, add all the ingredients except for zucchini and oil and then cook until sugar has dissolved.
2. Then place zucchini strips in a large bowl, pour in the mixture from the saucepan, toss until coated, and then let it marinate for a minimum of 1 hour.

3. When ready to cook, switch on the oven, set it to 400 degrees F, and let it preheat.

4. Take a baking sheet, line it with a parchment sheet, grease with oil, arrange marinated zucchini strips on it, and then bake for 10 minutes.

5. Then flip the zucchini, continue cooking for 4 minutes and then let cool completely.

6. Serve straight away.

16. Vegan Veggie Fritters

Serving: 2

Cooking time: 10 minutes;

Preparation time: 10 minutes;

Nutritional Info: 281.5 Cal; 15.2 g Fats; 13.8 g Protein; 26.2 g Carb; 5 g Fiber;

Ingredients:

- 1 cup chickpea flour
- 200g mushrooms, chopped
- 1 medium green bell pepper, cored, chopped
- 1 tablespoon onion powder
- 2 medium white onions, peeled, chopped

Extra:

- 1 teaspoon of sea salt
- 1 tablespoon oregano
- 1/8 teaspoon cayenne pepper
- 1 tablespoon grapeseed oil
- 1 tablespoon basil leaves, chopped
- ½ cup spring water

Directions

1. Put the vegetables in a bowl, add all the seasonings, basil and oregano, stir until mixed, and then let the mixture rest for 5 minutes.

2. Add chickpea flour, stir until mixed and then stir in water until well combined and smooth.
3. Take a large skillet pan, place it over medium heat, add oil and when hot, ladle vegetable mixture in it in portions, press down each portion, and then cook for 3 to 4 minutes per side until cooked and golden brown.
4. Serve straight away.

17. Chickpea and Mushroom Curry

Serving: 2

Cooking time: 12 minutes;

Preparation time: 5 minutes;

Nutritional Info: 194.7 Cal; 8.5 g Fats; 5.8 g Protein; 25.7 g Carb; 5.4 g Fiber;

Ingredients:

- 1 cup cooked chickpea
- 1 small white onion, peeled, diced
- ½ of medium green bell pepper, cored, chopped
- 1 cup diced mushrooms
- 8 cherry tomatoes, chopped

Extra:

- ½ teaspoon salt
- ¼ teaspoon cayenne pepper
- 1 teaspoon grapeseed oil

Directions

1. Take a medium skillet pan, place it over medium heat, add oil and when hot, add onion, tomatoes, and bell pepper and then cook for 2 minutes.
2. Add chickpeas and mushrooms, season with and cayenne pepper, stir until combined, and switch heat to medium-low level and then simmer for 10 minutes until cooked, covering the pan with its lid.
3. Serve straight away.

18. Vegetable Low Mein

Serving: 2

Cooking time: 10 minutes;

Preparation time: 5 minutes;

Nutritional Info: 330 Cal; 11 g Fats; 10 g Protein; 48 g Carb; 4 g Fiber;

Ingredients:

- 2 cups cooked spelt noodles
- ½ of medium green bell pepper, cored, sliced
- ½ of medium red bell pepper, cored, sliced
- 1 medium white onion, cored, sliced
- ½ cup sliced mushrooms

Extra:

- 2/3 teaspoon salt
- ¼ teaspoon onion powder
- 1/3 teaspoon cayenne pepper
- 1 key lime juiced
- 1 tablespoon sesame oil

Directions

1. Take a large skillet pan, place it over medium heat, add oil and when hot, add all the vegetables and cook for 3 to 5 minutes until a tender crisp forms.

2. Add all the spices, drizzle with lime juice, stir until mixed, and then cook for 1 minute.

3. Add noodles, toss until well mixed and then cook for 2 to 3 minutes until hot.

4. Serve straight away.

19. Spiced Okra Curry

Serving: 2

Cooking time: 10 minutes;

Preparation time: 5 minutes;

Nutritional Info: 137 Cal; 8.4 g Fats; 4 g Protein; 15 g Carb; 5.6 g Fiber;

Ingredients:

- 1 ½ cup okra
- 8 cherry tomatoes, chopped
- 1 medium onion, peeled, sliced
- ¾ cup vegetable broth, homemade

Extra:

- 6 teaspoons spice mix
- ¼ teaspoon salt
- ½ tablespoon grapeseed oil
- ¼ teaspoon cayenne pepper
- ¾ cup tomato sauce, alkaline
- 6 tablespoons soft-jelly coconut milk

Directions

1. Take a large skillet pan, place it over medium heat, add oil and warm, add onion, and then cook for 5 minutes until golden brown.
2. Add spice mix, add remaining ingredients into the pan except for okra, stir until mixed, and then bring the mixture to a simmer.

3. Add okra, stir until mixed, and then cook for 10 to 15 minutes over medium-low heat setting until cooked.
4. Serve straight away.

20. Baked Portobello Mushrooms

Serving: 2

Cooking time: 30 minutes;

Preparation time: 10 minutes;

Nutritional Info: 72 Cal; 2 g Fats; 6 g Protein; 10 g Carb; 2 g Fiber;

Ingredients:

- 2 caps of Portobello mushrooms, destemmed
- 2/3 teaspoon minced onion
- 2/3 teaspoon minced sage
- 2/3 teaspoon thyme
- 2/3 tablespoon key lime juice

Extra:

- 2 tablespoons alkaline soy sauce

Directions

1. Switch on the oven, then set it to 400 degrees F and let it preheat.
2. Take a baking dish and then arrange mushroom caps in it, cut side up.
3. Take a small bowl, place the remaining ingredients in it, stir until mixed, brush the mixture over inside and outside mushrooms, and then let them marinate for 15 minutes.
4. Bake the mushrooms for 30 minutes, flipping halfway, and then serve.

21. Kale and Sprouts Salad

Serving: 2

Preparation time: 5 minutes; Cooking time: 0 minutes;

Nutritional Info: 179.2 Cal; 14.1 g Fats; 3.7 g Protein; 13.5 g Carb; 6.1 g Fiber;

Ingredients:

- 2 cups kale leaves
- 1 cup sprouts
- 1 cup cherry tomato
- ½ of avocado, peeled, pitted, diced
- 1 key lime, juiced

Extra:

- 1 teaspoon agave syrup
- ½ tablespoon olive oil
- 1/8 teaspoon cayenne pepper

Directions

1. Take a small bowl, place lime juice in it, add oil and agave syrup and then stir until mixed.
2. Take a salad bowl, place remaining ingredients in it, drizzle with the lime juice mixture and then toss until mixed.
3. Serve straight away.

22. Chard and Lime Pasta

Serving: 2

Cooking time: 5 minutes;

Preparation time: 5 minutes;

Nutritional Info: 224 Cal; 7 g Fats; 7 g Protein; 33 g Carb; 2 g Fiber;

Ingredients:

- 1 head of Swiss chard, cut into ½-inch pieces
- 1 cup spelt pasta, cooked
- 2 green onions, sliced
- ¼ cup cilantro
- 1 key lime, juiced, zested

Extra:

- ¼ teaspoon salt
- ¼ teaspoon cayenne pepper
- 1 tablespoon olive oil

Directions

1. Take a large skillet pan, place it over medium heat, add oil and when hot, add chard pieces and then cook for 4 minutes or more until wilted.
2. Remove pan from heat, transfer chards to a large bowl, add remaining ingredients and then toss until combined.
3. Serve straight away.

23. Creamy Squash Soup

Serving: 2

Cooking time: 25 minutes;

Preparation time: 5 minutes;

Nutritional Info: 183 Cal; 14.4 g Fats; 1.9 g Protein; 13.4 g Carb; 2.7 g Fiber;

Ingredients:

- ½ of medium white onion, peeled, cubed
- 2 cups cubed squash
- ¼ cup basil leaves
- ½ cup soft-jelly coconut cream

Extra:

- 1/8 teaspoon sea salt
- 1/8 teaspoon cayenne pepper
- 1 tablespoon grapeseed oil
- 1 cup vegetable broth, homemade

Directions

1. Take a medium saucepan, place it over medium heat, add oil and when hot, add onion, and then cook for 5 minutes or until softened.
2. Add squash, cook for 10 minutes until golden and begin to soften, pour in the vegetable broth, season with salt and pepper and then bring the soup to boil.

3. Switch heat to medium level and then simmer the soup for 10 minutes until squash turns very soft.
4. Remove pan from heat, puree it by using a stick blender until smooth, and then garnish with basil.
5. Serve straight away.

24. Creamy Mushroom Soup

Serving: 2

Cooking time: 20 minutes;

Preparation time: 5 minutes;

Nutritional Info: 100 Cal; 2 g Fats; 2 g Protein; 18 g Carb; 2 g Fiber;

Ingredients:

- 2 cups baby Bella mushrooms, diced
- ½ cup diced red onions
- 1 cup vegetable broth
- 1 ½ cups soft-jelly coconut milk

Extra:

- ½ teaspoon of sea salt
- ¼ teaspoon cayenne pepper
- 2 teaspoons grapeseed oil

Directions

1. Take a medium saucepan, place it over medium-high heat, add oil and when hot, add onion, mushrooms, season with salt and pepper, and then cook for 3 to 4 minutes until vegetables turn tender.
2. Then add soy sauce, pour in milk and broth, stir until mixed and bring it to a boil.
3. Switch heat to medium-low level and then simmer the soup for 15 minutes until thickened to the desired level.
4. Serve straight away.

25. Onion Soup

Serving: 2

Cooking time: 35 minutes;

Preparation time: 5 minutes;

Nutritional Info: 76 Cal; 2.1 g Fats; 2.3 g Protein; 13.1 g Carb; 2.5 g Fiber;

Ingredients:

- 2 large white onions, peeled, sliced
- ½ cup cubed squash
- 1 sprig of thyme
- 1 tablespoon grapeseed oil
- 2 cups spring water

Extra:

- ½ teaspoon salt
- ¼ teaspoon cayenne pepper

Directions

1. Take a medium pot, place it over medium heat, add oil and when hot, add onion and cook for 10 minutes.
2. Add thyme sprig, switch heat to the low level and then cook onions for 15 to 20 minutes until soft, covering the pan with its lid.
3. Add remaining ingredients, stir until mixed and simmer for 5 minutes.
4. Ladle soup into bowls and then serve.

26. Roasted Squash and Apples

Serving: 2

Cooking time: 35 minutes;

Preparation time: 10 minutes;

Nutritional Info: 126.4 Cal; 4.9 g Fats; 1.1 g Protein; 22.2 g Carb; 5.1 g Fiber;

Ingredients:

- 1 ½ pounds butternut squash, peeled, deseeded, cut into chunks
- 2 apples, cored, cut into ½-inch pieces
- 2 tablespoons agave syrup
- 1/2 teaspoon sea salt

Extra:

- 2 tablespoons grapeseed oil

Directions

1. Switch on the oven, then set it to 375 degrees F and let it preheat.
2. Meanwhile, take a baking sheet and then spread squash pieces on it.
3. Take a small bowl, pour in oil, stir in salt and allspice until mixed, and then drizzle over squash pieces.
4. Cover the pan with foil and then bake for 20 minutes.
5. Meanwhile, place apple pieces in a medium bowl, drizzle with agave syrup, and then toss until coated.

6. When squash has baked, unwrap the baking sheet, spoon into the bowl containing the apple and then stir until mixed.

7. Spread apple-squash mixture evenly on the baking sheet and then continue baking for 15 minutes.

8. Serve straight away.

27. Mushroom Steak

Serving: 2

Cooking time: 10 minutes;

Preparation time: 10 minutes;

Nutritional Info: 302 Cal; 18 g Fats; 2 g Protein; 27 g Carb; 3 g Fiber;

Ingredients:

- 2 portabella mushroom caps, 1/8-inch thick sliced
- ½ cup sliced green bell peppers
- ½ cup sliced white onions
- ½ cup sliced red bell peppers
- ¼ cup alkaline sauce

Extra:

- ½ teaspoon of sea salt
- ½ tablespoon onion powder
- ½ teaspoon dried oregano
- ½ teaspoon dried thyme
- ½ tablespoon grapeseed oil
- 2 spelt flatbreads, toasted

Directions

1. Take a medium bowl, place sauce in it, add all the seasoning, and then whisk until combined.

2. Add mushroom slices, toss until coated, and then let them marinate for a minimum of 30 minutes, tossing halfway.

3. Then take a pan, place it over medium-high heat, add oil and when hot, add onion and pepper and cook for 3 to 5 minutes until tender-crisp.

4. Add mushroom slices, stir until mixed and continue cooking for 5 minutes.

5. Distribute vegetables evenly between flatbread, roll them, and then serve.

28. Chayote Mushroom Stew

Serving: 2

Cooking time: 40 minutes;

Preparation time: 10 minutes;

Nutritional Info: 173 Cal; 9 g Fats; 2 g Protein; 20 g Carb; 2 g Fiber;

Ingredients:

- 2/3 cup chayote squash cubes
- 1 cups sliced mushrooms
- 1/3 cup diced white onions
- ½ cup chickpea flour
- 1/3 cup vegetable broth, homemade

Extra:

- 1/3 tablespoon onion powder
- 2/3 teaspoon sea salt
- 2/3 teaspoon dried basil
- 1/3 teaspoon crushed red pepper
- 2 cups spring water
- ½ tablespoon grapeseed oil
- 1/3 cup hemp milk, homemade

Directions

1. Take a medium pot, place it over medium-high heat, add oil and when hot, add onion and mushroom, and then cook for 5 minutes.

2. Switch heat to medium level, pour in 1 cup water, milk, and broth, add chayote and all the seasoning, stir until mixed, and then bring it to a simmer, covering the pan with a lid.

3. Pour remaining water into a food processor, add chickpea flour, pulse until blended, add to the pot and then stir until mixed.

4. Switch heat to the low level, simmer for 30 minutes, and then serve.

29. Veggie Lettuce Wraps

Serving: 2

Cooking time: 0 minutes;

Preparation time: 10 minutes;

Nutritional Info: 155 Cal; 10.5 g Fats; 4.8 g Protein; 13.2 g Carb; 3.5 g Fiber;

Ingredients:

- ½ cup cherry tomatoes, halved
- 1 avocado, peeled, pitted, sliced
- ½ cup sprouts
- ½ of medium white onion, peeled, sliced
- 2 large lettuce leaves

Extra:

- 2 tablespoons key lime juice
- ½ tablespoon raisins
- ¼ teaspoon salt
- 1/8 teaspoon cayenne pepper

Directions

1. Take a small bowl, add lime juice, add salt and pepper and then stir until mixed.
2. Take a medium bowl, place all the vegetables in it except for lettuce, drizzle with the lime juice mixture and then toss until mixed.

3. Place lettuce leaves on a plate, top with half of the vegetable mixture, and then roll it tightly.

4. Repeat with the other lettuce wrap and then serve.

30. Vegan Rib Roast

Serving: 2

Cooking time: 15 minutes;

Preparation time: 10 minutes;

Nutritional Info: 108 Cal; 0.6 g Fats; 6 g Protein; 18 g Carb; 3 g Fiber;

Ingredients:

- 2 caps of Portobello mushrooms, ½ -inch thick sliced
- 1 teaspoon of sea salt
- ½ cup Alkaline Barbecue Sauce
- 1 teaspoon onion powder
- ¼ cup spring water

Extra:

- ½ teaspoon cayenne pepper
- 1 tablespoon grapeseed oil

Directions

1. Place mushroom slices in a container with a lid, add BBQ sauce, all the seasoning, and water, cover with a lid, and then shake until coated.
2. Place the container into the refrigerator and then let it marinate for a minimum of 6 hours, shaking every 2 hours.
3. When ready to cook, take a griddle pan, place it over medium-high heat, brush with oil and let it preheat.
4. Thread three slices of mushrooms in a skewer, then arrange these skewers on the pan and then cook for 15 minutes, flipping every 3 minutes.
5. Serve straight away.

31. Zucchini Linguine

Serving: 2

Cooking time: 8 minutes;

Preparation time: 10 minutes;

Nutritional Info: 284 Cal; 23.6 g Fats; 5.7 g Protein; 18.8 g Carb; 9.7 g Fiber;

Ingredients:

- 2 zucchinis, spiralized
- ½ cup sliced mushrooms
- ½ teaspoon dried thyme
- ½ cup alkaline Avocado sauce
- ¼ cup chopped cilantro

Extra:

- 1/3 teaspoon salt
- 1/8 teaspoon cayenne pepper
- 1 tablespoon grapeseed oil
- ½ teaspoon dried oregano

Directions

1. Take a skillet pan, place it over medium heat, add oil and when hot, add mushrooms and cilantro and then cook for 3 to 5 minutes until tender.

2. Add avocado sauce, season with salt, pepper, oregano, and thyme, stir until mixed and cook for 1 to 2 minutes until warmed.

3. Place zucchini noodles in a large bowl, drizzle with some oil, and then toss until well coated.

4. Add avocado mixture, toss until combined, and then serve.

32. Butternut Pumpkin Soup

Serving: 2

Cooking time: 15 minutes;

Preparation time: 5 minutes;

Nutritional Info: 133.3 Cal; 4.8 g Fats; 2.1 g Protein; 23.6 g Carb; 1.3 g Fiber;

Ingredients:

- 2 medium butternut squash, peeled, deseeded, chopped
- 1 medium white onion, peeled, chopped
- 2 cups soft-jelly coconut milk

Extra:

- 2/3 teaspoon sea salt
- 1 cup spring water

Directions

1. Take a large saucepan, place it over medium-high heat, pour in water, and then bring it to a boil.
2. Stir in salt and add vegetables and then cook for 5 to 10 minutes until vegetables turn tender.
3. Remove pan from heat, add milk and then puree by using an immersion blender until smooth.
4. Serve straight away.

33. Spiced Mushroom Bowl

Serving: 2

Cooking time: 10 minutes;

Preparation time: 5 minutes;

Nutritional Info: 186 Cal; 3.4 g Fats; 2.1 g Protein; 36.7 g Carb; 3.5 g Fiber;

Ingredients:

- 1 ½ cup sliced mushrooms
- 8 cherry tomatoes, chopped
- 1 medium onion, peeled, sliced
- ¾ cup vegetable broth, homemade

Extra:

- 6 teaspoons spice mix
- ¼ teaspoon salt
- ½ tablespoon grapeseed oil
- ¼ teaspoon cayenne pepper
- ¾ cup tomato sauce, alkaline
- 6 tablespoons soft-jelly coconut milk

Directions

1. Take a large skillet pan, place it over medium heat, add oil and warm, add onion, and then cook for 5 minutes until golden brown.

2. Add spice mix, add remaining ingredients into the pan except for okra, stir until mixed, and then bring the mixture to a simmer.
3. Add mushrooms, stir until mixed, and then cook for 10 to 15 minutes over medium-low heat setting until cooked.
4. Serve straight away.

34. Chickpea and Kale Curry

Serving: 2

Cooking time: 10 minutes;

Preparation time: 5 minutes;

Nutritional Info: 522 Cal; 38 g Fats; 15 g Protein; 26 g Carb; 8 g Fiber;

Ingredients:

- 2 cups cooked chickpeas
- 2/3 teaspoon salt
- 1 cup Kale leaves
- 2/3 cup soft-jelly coconut cream
- 2 tablespoons grapeseed oil

Extra:

- 1/3 teaspoon cayenne pepper

Directions

1. Switch on the oven, then set it to 425 degrees F and let it preheat.
2. Then take a medium baking sheet, spread chickpeas on it, drizzle with 1 tablespoon oil, sprinkle with all the seasonings and then bake for 15 minutes until roasted.
3. Then take a frying pan, place it over medium heat, add remaining oil and when hot, add kale and cook for 5 minutes.
4. Add roasted chickpeas, pour in the cream, stir until mixed and then simmer for 4 minutes, squashing chickpeas slightly.
5. Serve straight away.

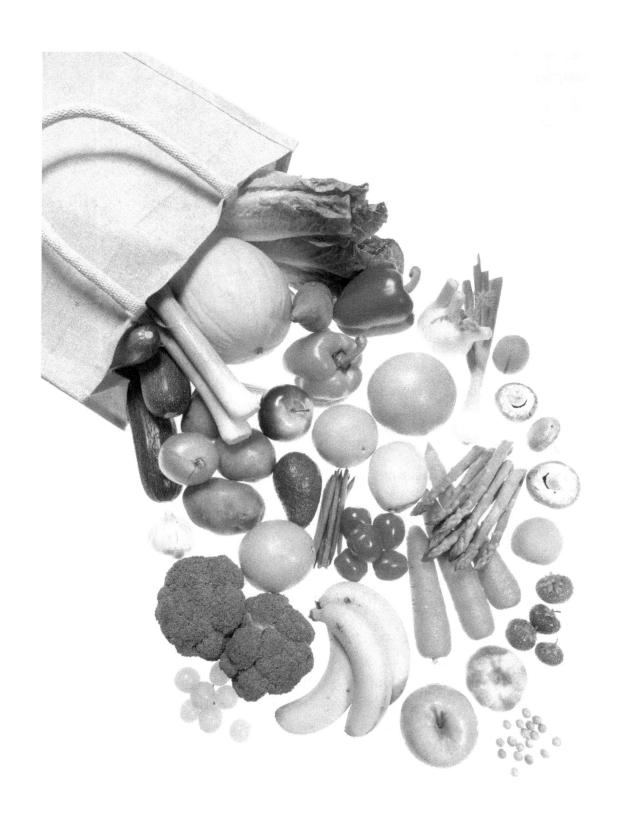

SOUPS, STEWS AND SAUCES

1. **Zoodle Vegetable Soup**

Serving: 2

Cooking time: 12 minutes;

Preparation time: 5 minutes;

Nutritional Info: 265 Cal; 2 g Fats; 4 g Protein; 57 g Carb; 13.6 g Fiber;

Ingredients:

- ½ of onion, peeled, cubed
- ½ of green bell pepper, chopped
- ½ of zucchini, grated
- 4 ounces sliced mushrooms, chopped
- ½ cup cherry tomatoes

Extra:

- ¼ cup basil leaves
- 1 pack of spelt noodles, cooked
- ¼ teaspoon salt
- 1/8 teaspoon cayenne pepper
- ½ of key lime, juiced
- 1 tablespoon grapeseed oil
- 2 cups spring water

Directions

1. Take a medium saucepan, place it over medium heat, add oil and when hot, add onion and then cook for 3 minutes or more until tender.

2. Add cherry tomatoes, bell pepper, and mushrooms, stir until mixed, and then continue cooking for 3 minutes until soft.

3. Add grated zucchini, season with salt, cayenne pepper, pour in the water and then bring the mixture to a boil.

4. Then switch heat to the low level, add cooked noodles and then simmer the soup for 5 minutes.

5. When done, ladle soup into two bowls, top with basil leaves, drizzle with lime juice and then serve.

2. Cucumber and Basil Gazpacho

Serving: 2

Preparation time: 5 minutes; Cooking time: 0 minutes;

Nutritional Info: 190 Cal; 15 g Fats; 4 g Protein; 15 g Carb; 6 g Fiber;

Ingredients:

- 1 avocado, peeled, pitted, cold
- 1 cucumber, deseeded, unpeeled, cold
- ½ cup basil leaves, cold
- ½ of key lime, juiced
- 2 cups spring water, chilled

Extra:

- 1 ½ teaspoon sea salt

Directions

1. Pour the ingredients into a high-speed food processor or blender and then pulse until smooth.
2. Tip the soup into a medium bowl and then chill for a minimum of 1 hour.
3. Divide the soup evenly between two bowls, top with some more basil and then serve.

3. Spicy Soursop and Zucchini Soup

Serving: 2

Cooking time: 45 minutes;

Preparation time: 5 minutes;

Nutritional Info: 224 Cal; 5 g Fats; 5.8 g Protein; 38.1 g Carb; 3.4 g Fiber;

Ingredients

- 1 cup chopped kale
- 2 Soursop leaves, rinsed, rip in half
- ½ cup summer squash cubes
- 1 cup chayote squash cubes
- ½ cup zucchini cubes

Extra:

- ½ cup wild rice
- ½ cup diced white onions
- 1 cup diced green bell peppers
- 2 teaspoons sea salt
- ½ tablespoon basil
- ¼ teaspoon cayenne pepper
- ½ tablespoon oregano
- 6 cups spring water

Directions

1. Take a medium pot, place it over medium-high heat, add soursop leaves, pour in 1 ½ cup water, and then boil for 15 minutes, covering the pan with a lid.

2. When done, remove eaves from the broth, switch heat to medium level, add remaining ingredients into the pot, stir until mixed, and then cook for 30 minutes or more until done.

3. Serve straight away.

4. Delicious Chickpea & Mushroom Bowl

Serving: 2

Cooking time: 10 minutes;

Preparation time: 5 minutes;

Nutritional Info: 242 Cal; 9 g Fats; 10 g Protein; 34 g Carb; 9 g Fiber;

Ingredients:

- 1 ½ cup cooked chickpeas
- 2 zucchinis, spiralized
- 4 small oyster mushrooms, destemmed, diced
- ¼ of white onion, peeled, chopped
- ¼ of red bell pepper, cored, chopped

Extra:

- 1/3 teaspoon sea salt; 1 teaspoon dried basil
- ¼ teaspoon cayenne pepper; 1 teaspoon dried oregano
- 1 tablespoon grapeseed oil
- 2 ½ cups vegetable broth, homemade

Directions

1. Take a medium pot, place it over medium-high heat, add oil and when hot, add red pepper, onion, and mushrooms, season with salt and cayenne pepper, and then cook for 5 minutes until tender.

2. Switch heat to medium-low level, add remaining ingredients except for zucchini noodles, stir until mixed, and then simmer the soup for 15 to 20 minutes.

3. Then add zucchini noodles into the pan, stir until mixed, and then cook for 1 minute or more until thoroughly warmed. Serve straight away.

5. Zoodle Chickpea Soup

Serving: 2

Cooking time: 25 minutes;

Preparation time: 5 minutes;

Nutritional Info: 184.5 Cal; 0.3 g Fats; 6.8 g Protein; 31 g Carb; 6 g Fiber;

Ingredients:

- ½ cup cooked, chickpeas
- ½ of a medium white onion, peeled, diced
- ½ of a large zucchini, chopped
- 1 cup kale leaves
- 1 cup squash cubes

Extra:

- ¾ teaspoon salt
- ¾ tablespoon chopped thyme, fresh
- ¾ tablespoon tarragon, fresh
- 2 cups vegetable broth, homemade
- 1 ½ cup spring water

Directions

1. Place a saucepan over medium-high heat, pour in the ¼ cup broth, add zucchini, onion, and thyme and then cook for 4 minutes.

2. Pour in the remaining broth and water, bring it to a boil, switch heat to the low level, and then simmer for 10 to 15 minutes until tender.

3. Add remaining ingredients, stir until mixed, and then continue cooking for 10 minutes or more until cooked.

4. Serve straight away.

6. Healthy Alkaline Green Soup

Serving: 2

Preparation time: 10 minutes; Cooking time: 10 minutes;

Nutritional Info: 129 Cal; 0.2 g Fats; 1.1 g Protein; 28 g Carb; 4.5 g Fiber;

Ingredients

- 2 cups leafy greens
- 1 small zucchini, sliced
- 1 small white onion, peeled, sliced
- 1 medium green bell pepper, cored, sliced
- 2 ½ cups spring water

Extra:

- ¾ teaspoon salt
- ¼ teaspoon cayenne pepper
- 1 teaspoon dried basil

Directions

1. Take a medium pot, place it over medium heat, add all the ingredients, stir until mixed, and then cook for 5 to 10 minutes until the vegetables turn tender-crisp.
2. Remove pot from heat, puree the soup by using an immersion blender and then serve.

7. Kamut Squash Soup

Serving: 2

Cooking time: 32 minutes;

Preparation time: 5 minutes;

Nutritional Info: 348.8 Cal; 8.8 g Fats; 11.3 g Protein; 57.2 g Carb; 7.8 g Fiber;

Ingredients:

- 6 tablespoons Kamut berries
- 1 cup chopped white onion
- ½ cup chopped squash
- ½ cup cooked chickpeas
- 1 cup vegetable broth, homemade

Extra:

- ¼ teaspoon cayenne pepper
- ½ tablespoon chopped tarragon
- 1 bay leaf
- 1 teaspoon chopped thyme
- 1 tablespoon olive oil
- 1 cup spring water, boiling

Directions

1. Place Kamut in a small bowl, pour in the boiling water, and let it stand for 30 minutes.

2. Then take a medium pot, place it over medium heat, add oil and when hot, add onion, stir in thyme and tarragon and then cook for 5 minutes until tender.

3. Drain Kamut, add to the pot, add bay leaves, pour in the vegetable broth, and then bring it to boil.

4. Cover the pot and subject it to heat for about 20 to 30 minutes, then stir in cayenne pepper and cook for 5 minutes.

5. Remove bay leaf, add chickpeas, and then cook for 2 minutes.

6. Serve straight away.

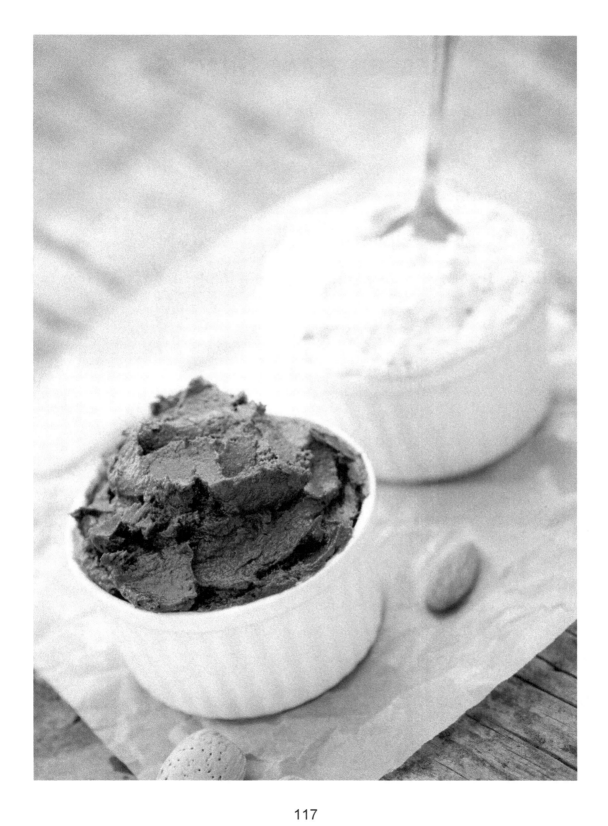

DESSERTS AND SNACKS

1.   **Alkaline Peach Muffin**

Serving: 2

Cooking time: 15 minutes;

Preparation time: 10 minutes;

Nutritional Info: 76.1 Cal; 3.3 g Fats; 0.9 g Protein; 14.3 g Carb; 0.9 g Fiber;

Ingredients:

- 2/3 cup spelt flour
- ½ of peach, chopped
- 1 teaspoon mashed burro banana
- 2/3 tablespoons chopped walnuts
- 6 ½ tablespoons walnut milk, homemade

Extra:

- 1/16 teaspoon salt
- 2 2/3 tablespoon date sugar
- 2/3 tablespoon spring water, warmed
- 2/3 teaspoon key lime juice

Directions

1. Switch on the oven, then set it to 400 degrees F and let it preheat.

2. Meanwhile, peel the peach, cut it in half, remove the pit and then cut one half of the peach in ½-inch pieces, reserving the other half of the peach for later use.

3. Take a medium bowl, pour in the milk, and then whisk in mashed burro banana and lime juice until well combined.

4. Take a separate medium bowl, place flour in it, add salt and date sugar, stir until mixed, whisk in milk mixture until smooth, and then fold in peaches until mixed.

5. Take four silicone muffin cups, grease them with oil, fill them evenly with the prepared batter and then sprinkle walnuts on top.

6. Bake the muffins for 10 to 15 minutes until the top is nicely golden brown and inserted toothpick into each muffin comes out clean.

7. When done, let muffins cool for 10 minutes and then serve.

2.   Nutty Brown Energy Balls

Serving: 2

Cooking time: 0 minutes;

Preparation time: 10 minutes;

Nutritional Info: 119 Cal; 8 g Fats; 2 g Protein; 10 g Carb; 1 g Fiber;

Ingredients:

- ¼ cup blueberries
- ¼ cup dried dates
- 1 cup soft-jelly coconut, shredded
- ¼ cup walnuts
- ½ teaspoon date sugar

Extra:

- ½ tablespoon agave syrup
- 1/16 teaspoon salt

Directions

1. Place walnuts in a food processor and then pulse until the mixture resembles a fine powder.
2. Then add berries, coconut, date sugar and dates, pulse until just mixed and then slowly blend in agave syrup until the soft paste comes together.
3. Spoon the mixture into a medium bowl, chill it for a minimum of 30 minutes and then roll the mixture into balls, 1 tablespoon of mixture per ball.
4. Roll the balls into some more coconut and then serve.

3. Flying Raspberry Energy Balls

Serving: 2

Preparation time: 5 minutes; Cooking time: 0 minutes;

Nutritional Info: 123 Cal; 8 g Fats; 1 g Protein; 11 g Carb; 2 g Fiber;

Ingredients:

- ½ cup raspberries
- 5 dates
- 1/16 teaspoon sea salt
- 1/3 cup walnuts
- 1 ½ cup soft-jelly coconut, shredded

Directions

1. Plug in a high-speed food processor or blender and add all the ingredients in its jar.
2. Cover the jar with its lid and then pulse for 40 to 60 seconds until well combined.
3. Shape the mixture into balls by using wet hands, 1 tablespoon of mixture per ball, place the balls on the tray, and let them freeze for a minimum of 30 minutes.
4. Serve straight away.

4.   Zucchini Bread Pancakes

Serving: 2

Cooking time: 8 minutes;

Preparation time: 10 minutes;

Nutritional Info: 130 Cal; 4 g Fats; 3 g Protein; 21 g Carb; 3 g Fiber;

Ingredients:

- 1 cup spelt flour
- ½ cup grated zucchini
- ¼ cup chopped walnuts
- 1 cup walnut milk, homemade

Extra:

- 1 tablespoon date sugar
- 1 tablespoon grapeseed oil

Directions

1. Take a medium bowl, place flour in it, add date sugar, and then stir until mixed.
2. Add mashed burro banana and milk in it, whisk until smooth batter comes together, and then fold in nuts and zucchini until just mixed.
3. Take a large skillet pan, place it over medium-high heat, add oil and when hot, pour the batter in it in portion and then shape each portion into a pancake.
4. Cook the pancake separately for 3 to 4 minutes per side and then serve.

5. Chickpea Nuggets

Serving: 2

Cooking time: 30 minutes;

Preparation time: 10 minutes;

Nutritional Info: 291.6 Cal; 3.9 g Fats; 19.9 g Protein; 26.8 g Carb; 3.4 g Fiber;

Ingredients:

- 2 cups cooked chickpeas
- ½ teaspoon salt
- 1 teaspoon onion powder
- 1/3 cup and 1 tablespoon bread crumbs

Directions

1. Switch on the oven, then set it to 350 degrees F and let it preheat.
2. Meanwhile, place chickpeas in a food processor and then pulse until crumbled.
3. Tip the chickpeas in a bowl, add remaining ingredients in it except for 1/3 cup of breadcrumbs and then stir until a chunky mixture comes together.
4. Shape the mixture into evenly sized balls, shape each ball into the nugget, arrange on a baking sheet greased with oil and then bake for 15 minutes per side until golden brown.
5. Serve straight away.

6. Special Spelt Banana Bread

Serving: 2

Cooking time: 20 minutes;

Preparation time: 10 minutes;

Nutritional Info: 186 Cal; 11.3 g Fats; 1.3 g Protein; 22 g Carb; 2 g Fiber;

Ingredients:

- 1/3 cup chopped walnuts
- 1 1/3 cup of burro banana
- 2/3 cup spelt flour
- 1/8 teaspoon salt
- ¼ cup agave syrup

Extra:

- 1 1/3 tablespoons olive oil

Directions

1. Switch on the oven, then set it to 350 degrees F and let it preheat.
2. Meanwhile, place the burro banana in a medium bowl, mash it by using a fork and then stir in oil and agave syrup until combined.
3. Take a separate medium bowl, place flour in it, add salt and nuts, stir until mixed, and then stir in the burro banana mixture until smooth.
4. Transfer the batter into a pan and bake for 20 minutes until firm and the top turn golden brown.

5. When done, let the bread cool for 10 minutes, then cut it into slices and serve.

7. Invigorating Sea Moss Pudding

Serving: 2

Preparation time: 5 minutes; Cooking time: 0 minutes;

Nutritional Info: 97.8 Cal; 0.5 g Fats; 0.7 g Protein; 23.4 g Carb; 2.8 g Fiber;

Ingredients:

- 2 burro bananas, peeled
- 2 cups blueberries
- 6 tablespoons of sea moss gel
- ½ cup spring Water

Directions

1. Plug in a high-speed food processor or blender and add all the ingredients in its jar except for water.
2. Cover the blender jar with its lid, pulse until smooth, and then slowly blend in water until thickened to the desired level.
3. Serve straight away.

8.   Delicious Avocado Tomato Toast

Serving: 2

Preparation time: 5 minutes; Cooking time: 0 minutes;

Nutritional Info: 189 Cal; 11 g Fats; 3 g Protein; 20 g Carb; 5.4 g Fiber;

Ingredients:

- 2 slices of spelt bread, toasted
- 1 avocado, peeled, pitted, mashed
- ½ cup cherry tomato halves
- ½ teaspoon salt
- 2 teaspoons key lime juice

Directions

1. Place avocado in a container, add lime juice and then mash until smooth.
2. Spread mashed avocado evenly on top of each toast and then scatter cherry tomatoes.
3. Sprinkle salt over tomatoes and then serve.

9. Tasty Rye Crackers

Serving: 2

Preparation time: 10 minutes; Cooking time: 10 minutes;

Nutritional Info: 81.2 Cal; 1.2 g Fats; 0.8 g Protein; 16.4 g Carb; 1.7 g Fiber;

Ingredients:

- 1 cup rye flour
- 1 teaspoon onion powder
- ½ teaspoon salt
- ½ teaspoon dried thyme
- ½ teaspoon dried basil

Extra:

- 2 tablespoons grapeseed oil
- 4 tablespoons spring water

Directions

1. Switch on the oven, then set it to 400 degrees F and let it preheat.
2. Meanwhile, place flour in a food processor, add all the seasonings and oil, and then pulse until combined.
3. Add water, pulse until the dough comes together, and then roll it into a ½-inch thick dough.
4. Use a cookie cutter of the desired shape to cut out the cookie, arrange them on a large baking sheet and then bake for 10 minutes until nicely browned.
5. Serve straight away.

10. Healthy Date Balls

Serving: 2

Preparation time: 5 minutes; Cooking time: 0 minutes;

Nutritional Info: 99.1 Cal; 5.3 g Fats; 2 g Protein; 13.5 g Carb; 2 g Fiber;

Ingredients:

- ¼ cup walnuts
- ½ cup dates, pitted
- ¼ cup sesame seeds
- ½ cup soft-jelly coconut, grated
- 2 tablespoons agave syrup

Extra:

- ¼ teaspoon of sea salt

Directions

1. Plug in a high-speed food processor or blender and add all the ingredients in its jar except for sesame seeds.
2. Cover the blender/container with its lid and then pulse for 20 seconds until well combined.
3. Tip the mixture into a bowl, shape it into even size balls and then roll each ball into sesame seeds.
4. Serve straight away.

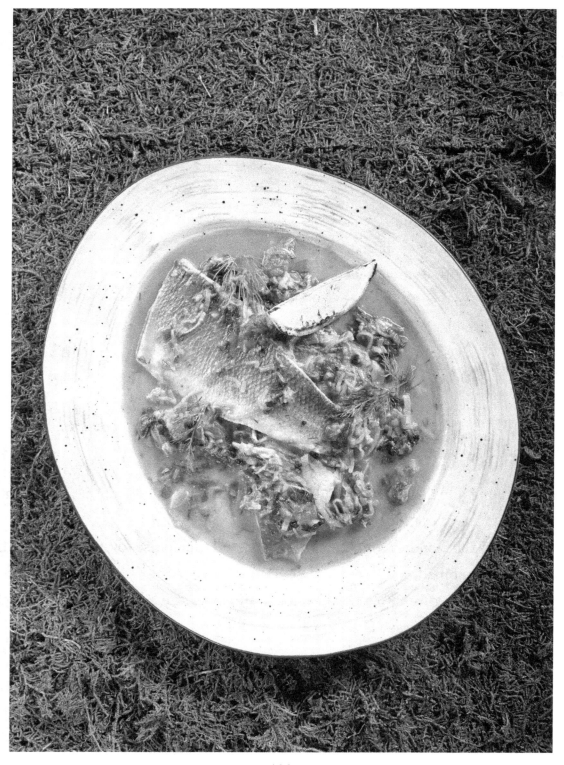

SEA MOSS RECIPES

1.   **Sea Moss Gel Recipe**

Serving: 2

Cooking time: 0 minutes;

Preparation time: 5 minutes;

Ingredients:

- 1 pack organic Irish sea moss
- 1/2 Cup Spring Water

Directions

1. Take a pack of sea moss and cut it into chunks.
2. Wash and soak in spring water for 6 hours.
3. Drain from water.
4. Plug in a high-speed food processor or blender and add the drained sea moss and water to its jar.
5. Cover the jar with its lid and then pulse for 40 to 60 seconds
6. until smooth.
7. Divide the gel between mason jars to be stored in the refrigerator, or
8. serve immediately.

2. Banana Mango Moss Recipe

Serving: 2

Preparation time: 5 minutes;

Cooking time: 0 minutes;

Ingredients:

- 1 burro banana, peeled
- ½ mango, peeled
- 1 mason jar sea moss gel
- 1 tablespoon green coconut water
- ½ cup hemp milk, homemade

Directions

1. Take out a jar of prepared sea moss gel.
2. Plug in a high-speed food processor or blender and add all the ingredients to its jar.
3. Cover the jar with its lid and then pulse for 40 to 60 seconds until smooth.
4. Divide the drink between two glasses and then serve.

3.   Creamy Sea Moss Milk Recipe

Serving: 2

Preparation time: 5 minutes;

Cooking time: 0 minutes;

Ingredients:

- 1 burro banana, peeled
- ½ cup dates
- 1 mason jar sea moss gel
- ½ cup walnut milk, homemade

Directions

1. Take out a jar of prepared sea moss gel.
2. Plug in a high-speed food processor or blender and add all the ingredients to its jar.
3. Cover the jar with its lid and then pulse for 40 to 60 seconds until smooth.
4. Divide the drink between two glasses and then serve.

4.   **Sea Moss Berry Shake**

Serving: 2

Preparation time: 5 minutes;

Cooking time: 0 minutes;

Ingredients:

- 1 burro banana, peeled
- ½ cup blueberries
- ½ cup raspberries
- ½ mason jar sea moss gel
- ½ cup hemp milk, homemade

Directions

1. Take out a jar of prepared sea moss gel.
2. Plug in a high-speed food processor or blender and add all the ingredients to its jar.
3. Cover the jar with its lid and then pulse for 40 to 60 seconds until smooth.
4. Divide the drink between two glasses and then serve.

5. Sunshine Sea Moss Drink

Serving: 2

Preparation time: 5 minutes;

Cooking time: 0 minutes;

Ingredients:

- 1 burro banana, peeled
- ½ mango, medium, peeled and chopped
- ½ mason jar sea moss gel
- ½ cup walnut milk (optional)

Directions

1. Take out a jar of prepared sea moss gel.
2. Plug in a high-speed food processor or blender and add all the ingredients to its jar.
3. Cover the jar with its lid and then pulse for 40 to 60 seconds until smooth.
4. Divide the drink between two glasses and then serve.

6. Alkaline Sea Moss Candy

Serving: 2

Preparation time: 5 minutes;

Cooking time: 0 minutes;

Ingredients:

- ½ cup raspberries
- ½ cup blackberries
- 1 avocado, destoned and peeled
- ½ jar sea moss gel
- ½ cup hemp milk
- 2 tablespoon date sugar (or as needed)

Directions

1. Take out a jar of prepared sea moss gel.
2. Plug in a high-speed food processor or blender and add all the ingredients to its jar.
3. Cover the jar with its lid and then pulse for 40 to 60 seconds until smooth.
4. Pour mixture into popsicle molds.
5. Freeze candy for 3 hours and serve.

7.   Blueberry Sea Moss Shake

Serving: 2

Preparation time: 5 minutes;

Cooking time: 0 minutes;

Ingredients:

- ½ cup blueberries
- 1 mason jar sea moss gel
- ½ cup hemp milk, (optional)
- 1 tablespoon date sugar

Directions

1. Take out a jar of prepared sea moss gel.
2. Plug in a high-speed food processor or blender and add all the ingredients to its jar.
3. Cover the jar with its lid and then pulse for 40 to 60 seconds until smooth.
4. Divide the drink between two glasses and then serve.

8. Fruity Sea Moss Recipe

Serving: 2

Preparation time: 5 minutes;

Cooking time: 0 minutes;

Ingredients:

- 1/3 pack dried fruit of choice
- 1 burro banana, peeled
- 1 mason jar sea moss gel
- ½ cup walnut milk, homemade

Directions

1. Take out a jar of prepared sea moss gel.
2. Plug in a high-speed food processor or blender and add all the ingredients to its jar.
3. Cover the jar with its lid and then pulse for 40 to 60 seconds until smooth.
4. Divide the drink between two glasses and then serve.

9. Avocado Creamy Moss Drink

Serving: 2

Preparation time: 5 minutes;

Cooking time: 0 minutes;

Ingredients

- 1 Avocado, destoned and peeled
- ½ cup raspberries
- 1 mason jar sea moss gel
- ½ cup walnut milk, homemade
- Handful dates

Directions

1. Take out a jar of prepared sea moss gel.
2. Plug in a high-speed food processor or blender and add all the ingredients to its jar.
3. Cover the jar with its lid and then pulse for 40 to 60 seconds until smooth.
4. Divide the drink between two glasses and then serve.

10. Banana Moss Recipe

Serving: 2

Preparation time: 5 minutes;

Cooking time: 0 minutes;

Ingredients

- 1 burro banana, peeled
- 1 mason jar sea moss gel
- 1 tablespoon date sugar
- ½ cup hemp milk, homemade

Directions

1. Take out a jar of prepared sea moss gel.
2. Plug in a high-speed food processor or blender and add all the ingredients to its jar.
3. Cover the jar with its lid and then pulse for 40 to 60 seconds until smooth.
4. Divide the drink between two glasses and then serve.

11. Berry Moss Drink

Serving: 2

Preparation time: 5 minutes;

Cooking time: 0 minutes;

Ingredients

- ½ cup strawberries
- 1 mason jar sea moss gel
- ½ cup hemp milk, homemade
- 1 tablespoon date sugar

Directions

1. Take out a jar of prepared sea moss gel.
2. Plug in a high-speed food processor or blender and add all the ingredients to its jar.
3. Cover the jar with its lid and then pulse for 40 to 60 seconds until smooth.
4. Divide the drink between two glasses and then serve.

12. Nutty Sea Moss Shake

Serving: 2

Preparation time: 5 minutes;

Cooking time: 0 minutes;

Ingredients

- 1 burro banana, peeled
- ½ cup dates
- ½ cup green coconut water
- 1 mason jar sea moss gel
- ½ cup hemp milk, homemade

Directions

1. Take out a jar of prepared sea moss gel.
2. Plug in a high-speed food processor or blender and add all the ingredients to its jar.
3. Cover the jar with its lid and then pulse for 40 to 60 seconds until smooth.
4. Divide the drink between two glasses and then serve.

13. Apple Sea Moss Delight

Serving: 2

Preparation time: 5 minutes;

Cooking time: 0 minutes;

Ingredients

- 1 Apple, chopped
- ½ banana, peeled
- 1 mason jar sea moss gel
- ½ cup walnut milk, homemade

Directions

1. Take out a jar of prepared sea moss gel.
2. Plug in a high-speed food processor or blender and add all the ingredients to its jar.
3. Cover the jar with its lid and then pulse for 40 to 60 seconds until smooth.
4. Divide the drink between two glasses and then serve.

14. Nutty Irish Moss Milkshake

Serving: 2

Preparation time: 5 minutes;

Cooking time: 0 minutes;

Ingredients:

- 1 burro banana, peeled
- ½ cup walnuts
- 1 mason jar sea moss gel
- ½ cup hemp milk, homemade
- 2 tablespoons date sugar

Directions

1. Take out a jar of prepared sea moss gel.
2. Plug in a high-speed food processor or blender and add all the ingredients to its jar.
3. Cover the jar with its lid and then pulse for 40 to 60 seconds until smooth.
4. Divide the drink between two glasses and then serve.

15. Peachy Moss Drink Recipe

Serving: 2

Preparation time: 5 minutes;

Cooking time: 0 minutes;

Ingredients:

- 1 burro banana, peeled
- 1 peach, peeled
- ½ cup raspberries
- 1 mason jar sea moss gel
- 1 tablespoon date sugar
- ½ cup hemp milk, homemade

Directions

1. Take out a jar of prepared sea moss gel.
2. Plug in a high-speed food processor or blender and add all the ingredients to its jar.
3. Cover the jar with its lid and then pulse for 40 to 60 seconds until smooth.
4. Divide the drink between two glasses and then serve.

16. Banana Date Moss Drink

Serving: 2

Preparation time: 5 minutes;

Cooking time: 0 minutes;

Ingredients:

- 1 burro banana, peeled
- 1 cup dates
- 1 mason jar sea moss gel
- ½ cup hemp milk, homemade

Directions

1. Take out a jar of prepared sea moss gel.
2. Plug in a high-speed food processor or blender and add all the ingredients to its jar.
3. Cover the jar with its lid and then pulse for 40 to 60 seconds until smooth.
4. Divide the drink between two glasses and then serve.

17. Creamy Strawberry Jar

Serving: 2

Preparation time: 5 minutes;

Cooking time: 0 minutes;

Ingredients:

- 1 burro banana, peeled
- 1 cup strawberries
- ½ mason jar sea moss gel
- 1 cup hemp milk, homemade
- 1 tablespoon date sugar

Directions

1. Take out a jar of prepared sea moss gel.
2. Plug in a high-speed food processor or blender and add all the ingredients to its jar.
3. Cover the jar with its lid and then pulse for 40 to 60 seconds until smooth.
4. Divide the drink between two glasses and then serve.

18. Banana Date Sea Moss Shake

Serving: 2

Preparation time: 5 minutes;

Cooking time: 0 minutes;

Ingredients:

- 1 burro banana, peeled
- ½ cup dates
- 1 mason jar sea moss gel
- ½ cup hemp milk, homemade

Directions

1. Take out a jar of prepared sea moss gel.
2. Plug in a high-speed food processor or blender and add all the ingredients to its jar.
3. Cover the jar with its lid and then pulse for 40 to 60 seconds until smooth.
4. Divide the drink between two glasses and then serve.

19. Simple Sea Moss Recipe

Serving: 2

Preparation time: 5 minutes;

Cooking time: 0 minutes;

Ingredients:

- 1 mason jar sea moss gel
- 1 tablespoon date sugar
- ½ cup spring water

Directions

1. Take out a jar of prepared sea moss gel.
2. Plug in a high-speed food processor or blender and add all the ingredients to its jar.
3. Cover the jar with its lid and then pulse for 40 to 60 seconds until smooth.
4. Divide the drink between two glasses and then serve.

20. Berry Mix Moss Milk

Serving: 2

Preparation time: 5 minutes;

Cooking time: 0 minutes;

Ingredients

- 1 cup berry mix
- ½ mason jar sea moss gel
- ½ cup hemp milk (optional)

Directions

1. Take out a jar of prepared sea moss gel.
2. Plug in a high-speed food processor or blender and add all the ingredients to its jar.
3. Cover the jar with its lid and then pulse for 40 to 60 seconds until smooth.
4. Divide the drink between two glasses and then serve.

21. Sea Moss Coconut Drink

Serving: 2

Preparation time: 5 minutes;

Cooking time: 0 minutes;

Ingredients:

- ½ cup raspberries
- 1 mason jar sea moss gel
- ½ cup green coconut water
- 1 tablespoon date sugar (optional)

Directions

1. Take out a jar of prepared sea moss gel.
2. Plug in a high-speed food processor or blender and add all the ingredients to its jar.
3. Cover the jar with its lid and then pulse for 40 to 60 seconds until smooth.
4. Divide the drink between two glasses and then serve.

CPSIA information can be obtained
at www.ICGtesting.com
Printed in the USA
LVHW061117300621
690925LV00047B/1636